PRIMITIVE SURGERY

PRIMITIVE SURGERY

Skills Before Science

By

SPENCER L. ROGERS, Ph.D.

Research Anthropologist
San Diego Museum of Man
San Diego, California

Professor Emeritus of Anthropology
San Diego State University

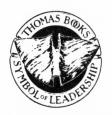

CHARLES C THOMAS • PUBLISHER
Springfield • Illinois • U.S.A.

Published and Distributed Throughout the World by

CHARLES C THOMAS • PUBLISHER

2600 South First Street

Springfield, Illinois 62717

© *1985 by* CHARLES C THOMAS • PUBLISHER

ISBN 0-398-05123-2

Library of Congress Catalog Card Number: 84-26910

With **THOMAS BOOKS** *careful attention is given to all details of manufacturing and design. It is the Publisher's desire to present books that are satisfactory as to their physical qualities and artistic possibilities and appropriate for their particular use.* THOMAS BOOKS *will be true to those laws of quality that assure a good name and good will.*

Printed in the United States of America
Q-R-3

Library of Congress Cataloging in Publication Data

Rogers, Spencer Lee, 1905-
    Primitive surgery.

    Bibliography: p.
    Includes indexes.
    1. Surgery, Primitive — History. I. Title.
[DNLM: 1. History of Medicine, Ancient.
2. Surgery — history. WO 11.1 R729p]
GN477.5.R63 1985   617.91'009'01   84-26910
ISBN 0-398-05123-2

TO THOSE prehistoric antecedent surgeons, who, without science or recorded tradition, first explored ways of relieving human suffering and restoring body functions through the manipulation of tissue.

ACKNOWLEDGMENTS

I WISH to acknowledge most cordially the assistance that I have received from Jane Bentley, the librarian of the San Diego Museum of Man. She has been most cooperative and resourceful in finding the documents that were involved in the materials here presented.

I also acknowledge the careful manuscript preparation on the part of Patricia Burton. Her skill and technique are most highly appreciated.

Spencer L. Rogers

CONTENTS

PRIMITIVE SURGERY

INTRODUCTION

THE SCOPE AND METHODS OF
PRE-SCIENTIFIC SURGERY

SURGERY is a unique area of technology. Man's own body becomes an artifact, something to be worked upon, manipulated and changed by human hands. The motives for applying operative skills to human body substance have been many, usually for a beneficial purpose to the subject, but not always. Much of surgery has been dedicated to the setting right of some derangement in body function, such as removing a foreign object embedded in the flesh or curing a headache, but there have been various other motives. Surgical operations have been performed on young healthy persons to promote well-being and longevity in later life. Operations have been for ritual reasons, such as circumcision and subincision, and also for judical reasons such as marking a slave and the punishment of a criminal, as cutting off an ear or removing a hand. Again considerable minor surgery has been performed for aesthetic reasons such as tatooing or scarification and piercing the lips, nose and ears. When surgery began is unknown but it could well have been back toward the dawn of culture.

The term "primitive" in the title of this work requires a brief explanation. The word is used to mean prescientific, an epoch of culture without recorded observations and organized knowledge, without experimentally derived data and tested hypotheses. It does not necessarily mean unskilled, irresponsible and ineffective. "Primitive" treatments, including folk medications and some surgical maneuvers by unlettered medicinemen, have undoubtedly ac-

MAP 1: MAJOR AREAS OF PRIMITIVE TREPHINING IN THE EASTERN HEMISPHERE

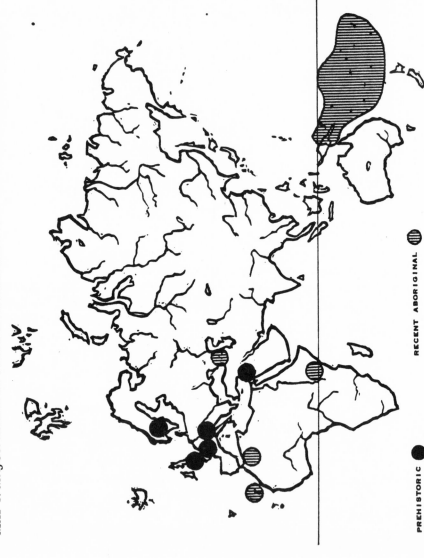

PREHISTORIC RECENT ABORIGINAL

MAP 2: PRIMITIVE TREPHINING IN THE WESTERN HEMISPHERE

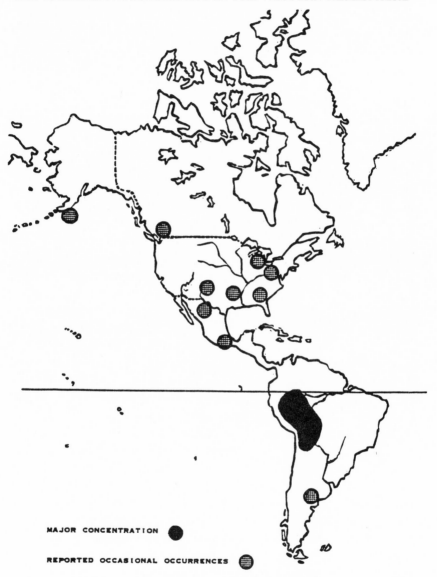

MAJOR CONCENTRATION

REPORTED OCCASIONAL OCCURRENCES

complished a considerable degree of healing in human history. What is attempted here is a review of the methods and, as far as possible, the doctrine and practices involved in surgical ministrations in a number of cultures of both hemispheres that were without scientific medicine. These include the early Greeks, the Romans, the early Britons, the Hindus, and also the aboriginal peoples of Africa, America, and Oceania.

In dealing with the development of surgery we can consider several aspects in both time and geography. First is our knowledge of the beginnings of the surgical craft among prehistoric peoples, mainly in Europe, Asia and north Africa. Evidences from the remote past consist essentially of bones and skulls, mainly skulls that show evidence of surgical operations. Secondly we have data from the classical cultures of Europe and north Africa, the Egyptians, Greeks and Romans. From these we have written records in the form of descriptions of surgical techniques and also some artistic portrayals of surgical instruments and operations, as well as some instruments that have been well preserved. A third source of data is in the reported observations of recent and living aboriginal peoples of Africa and Arabia, who during pre- and post-Christian times down to the present have developed medical traditions. A fourth area of importance includes peoples of the Americas before and shortly after the opening of aboriginal America to European contacts; also certain Oceanic Islanders. Each of these culture phases provides evidence that wil be discussed in turn.

We have three basic tasks before us. One is to review briefly the technology of surgery from its beginning as far as the data of archaeology make this possible. A second objective is to review the significant elements of surgical technology of the ancient literate cultures of Egypt, Greece and Rome. A third intention is to canvass the surgical methods of certain prescientific cultures, later historical and recent, that illustrate the approach of peoples who, without the background of scientific anatomy, physiology and pathology, have performed operations for various reasons.

By examining ancient and recent prescientific cultures an answer is sought for the fundamental question: Through what stages and by what transformations did the prescientific surgeon move toward the status of a scientific practitioner? From this overview it may be possible to note the groping of early surgeons toward a body of knowledge and theory of practice that eventually became the surgery of today.

In the beginning it is important to glance briefly at the range of surgical ministrations that various peoples have undertaken, with some reflections on the degree of technical proficiency required in these several areas (see table).

One important form of surgery involves no cutting of tissue, only the restoration of body elements that have been deranged through fractures or dislocations. *Manipulative surgery* includes mainly the reduction of fractures and dislocations, and depends largely on the knowledge and skill of the operator in bringing the body elements into their proper anatomical relationships. The operator usually makes no incisions, but through his knowledge of bones and joints and his skill in manipulation is able to restore the normal anatomical associations. He needs no profound theoretical background, but an understanding of skeletal anatomy of the region involved and a sense of the movements necessary to bring the distorted elements into their normal interconnections. He does need a measure of skill and strength, and sometimes ingenuity in designing a "luxation table" and in fitting splints, but no minute fingertip precision in muscular control.

Another level of surgery may be classed as *minor operative*. This has a wide range of apllications. It quite commonly involves the removal of some foreign object from the patient's body, such as an arrow point between his ribs or a thorn embedded in his foot. The doctor's role here is merely to remove the offending object, by seizing and pulling and often by making an incision in order to reach and release the item. Other minor operative measures include the incision of boils or pustules in order to evacuate fluid, and the cutting away of torn flesh from a wound. An entirely different area of practice is in the piercing or cutting of tissue for reasons other than curative. Ears have been pierced in order to fit them with rings or plugs, the nasal septum pierced in order to insert a nosepin; the body scarified or tatooed or the teeth drilled and filed to a point, all so that the mutilated person would conform to a culturally defined pattern or decoration or symbolism.

ASPECTS OF SURGERY WITH PARTICULAR REFERENCE TO PRESCIENTIFIC TECHNIQUES

Type	Examples	Instruments employed	Knowledge and skill involved
MANIPULATIVE SURGERY	Reduction of fractures and dislocations.	Hands and muscles of the operator; perhaps frames and "luxation tables"; some fitting of splints	Basic knowledge of joint anatomy; considerable manual skill and strength.
MINOR OPERATIVE SURGERY	Incision of boils and pustules, removal of embedded objects, debridement of wounds; piercing and cutting of skin for cosmetic, ritual or judicial reasons.	Knives of stone, bronze or iron, piercing instruments of stone, thorns or teeth, grinding stones for tooth mutilation.	Some knowledge of surficial anatomy of the region involved.
MAJOR OPERATIVE SURGERY	Amputation of legs, arms, hands; trephination of the skull, appendectomy, lithotomy, Caesarian section, lendectomy for cataracts.	A wide selection of knives, saws, scrapers, hemostats, probes, retractors, elevators, tenaculums, needles and sutures. Some of these were but crudely improvised before the working of metals.	A practical knowledge of the anatomy of the region involved; a high level of hand and finger dexterity; also the ability to sense the relationship of elements in three dimensional structures.

Judiciary and ritual surgery form a special category. Many peoples who have had little surgical knowledge or skill in dealing with problems that required treatment for body disorders, performed radical excisions and amputations either as ritual measures or as punishment for legal and ethical violations. However, among some peoples, notably those of Central Africa, body mutilation of any sort, including tooth extraction, was resisted because it would supposedly interfere with the future life of the person's ghost (Ackerknecht 1947: 39).

Major operative procedures bring into play another level of doctrine and skill. These operations may include the amputation of an arm or leg, or the removal of an inflamed gallbladder, the removal of an inflamed vermiform appendix, Caesarian section, the removal of cataracts from the eyes or trephining the skull. All these operations involve some theoretical understanding and a considerable degree of skill. The greater the surgeon's skill, the greater the patient's chance of recovery and return to normality, although a skillful operation may often have been followed by the death of the patient for various reasons unconnected with the specific surgical manipulation.

The nature of the surgeon's instruments is an interesting and important aspect of his technology. The operating equipment of the Stone Age surgeon is difficult to determine. He may have made some use of wood fibers and thorns for piercing and elevating devices, but his knives were undoubtedly for the most part of igneous rock capable of being chipped and flaked to a sharp working edge, although for some peoples shell may have been convenient and effective. Many flake tools have been found in Neolithic and earlier Stone Age sites. The problem here is that knives and scraper blades that could have been used for surgical purposes also could have been used for cutting leather, fleshing hides and numerous other utilitarian purposes, and cannot with assurance be characterized as surgical imlements. With the advent of metal technology, implements more specifically surgical were made and these can often be identified. Bronze and iron saws, retractors, forceps, tanaculums, probes and trocars are found in Greek and Roman archaeological sites and there is little doubt as to their purpose.

It can reasonably be postulated that a Stone Age surgeon sufficiently skilled to perform a number of exacting operations would also have been able to fabricate from wood, thorns, stone and shell, the basic apparatus that he needed in his professional activities. There is ample evidence that Palaeolithic and Neolithic craftsmen were expert in manipulating stone in making points, blades and figurines. They undoubtedly extended their technical activities to other media that have left no trace. Some of their capability could well have been employed in devising surgical implements from the variety of materials at their disposal.

As a final introductory note it should be stressed that the pre-scientific doctor was probably not only a surgical practitioner but also a medicine man. It is quite likely that in most cases his tissue manipulations were accompanied by boasts of supernatural powers and mythological references. He probably gave mystical reasons for the operations that he was about to perform and explained his surgical maneuvers as devices to expel evil spirit forces from his patient's body or to provide an entry for benign agencies. This aspect of surgery survived into the Middle Ages with references to astrology and horoscopes. Surgery has perhaps always been accompanied by a mystery that has provided it with a psychotherapeutic role.

In the following discussion the term surgery is interpreted to mean any intentional manipulation of human tissue, regardless of the motive. This includes more than surgery for healing purposes. Some cutting, piercing and slashing of the body is obviously done for reasons connected with ceremonial symbolism, decoration or punishment. Yet it is at times difficult to be certain as to which motivation applies. Scarification is at times associated with bloodletting as a form of healing or preventive therapy, yet it is also done for purely decorative or symbolic reasons. Since it is often difficult to interpret the thinking of ancient peoples and non-Westernized aborigines it has been decided in this work to include any cutting, puncturing, slashing or even chopping of the human body as surgical. It is conceded that at times the motives are often obvious but again more than one motive may be involved or the reason may be obscure. It has been considered best to avoid speculative and perhaps erroneous categorization and keep the definition broad and inclusive.

Throughout the following discussion many of the ethnographic descriptions are in the present tense. It is thoroughly understood that in most areas the aboriginal procedures have been completely or essentially supplanted by Western medical technology. Yet, since it is usually impossible to establish the time and degree of transition to Western healing practices, descriptions in most cases will be left in the present tense, which was applicable at the time they were first observed and reported.

CHAPTER 1

THE EARLIEST EVIDENCE

Surgery in Stone Age Europe and Asia

THERE IS no way of knowing when and where the earliest surgery was performed. Phases of superficial surgery were perhaps a part of the universal groping effort of human beings to deal with irregularities in their own conditions or those of other members of their community. This would include the digging out of splinters embedded in the skin, the piercing of blisters and boils and the removal of damaged tissue from wounds. The earliest possible evidence up to the present pertaining to surgery is the problematical indication of amputation of the right forearm of a Neanderthal skeleton, Shanidar I, found in the Zagros mountains of Iraq in 1957. This skeleton is probably 40,000 years old. The right arm from the humerus down is missing although the radius and ulna of the left arm were recovered. The implication is that the right forearm had either been severed in some type of accident or amputated (Stewart 1977: 128). The earliest body of evidence of major surgery now available is in the skulls recovered from Neolithic sites, mainly dating probably between 3000 B.C. and 2000 B.C.

There is possible evidence that trephination, or a crude skull opening operation antecedent to trephining, may have been performed prior to Neolithic times. A skull discovered at Taforalt, France, in a pre-Neolithic cultural level has an almost circular shaped depression in the left parietal bone that has been considered a primitive effort toward trephining (Dastugue 1959: 357-363).

Most of the prehistoric trephined skulls have been found in Western Europe and Asia (see Map 1). They show trephine openings which average around 4 centimeters across. Some indicate that the patient died during or shortly after the operation, but many give evidence of surviving for some time, even to be trephined several times (Ruffer 1918-1919: 93-94). Well over half show healing after the surgery. The trephining operation, which is technically exacting, may not have been the only surgical achievement known to prehistoric peoples since soft tissue operations would have left no trace. From the trephined skulls now recovered we have data on the trephine operation and know that this aspect of surgery flourished in a wide geographic area in the prehistoric past and also we have evidence of the methods used and the frequency of healing. We have only speculations as to the reasons for performing the operation but there have been many interesting theories.

The art of performing successfully the trephine operation was often practiced during the New Stone age in Europe and parts of Asia, later becoming known in Africa, Oceania and the New World. By ethnographic inference based on the number of known cases, Western Europe would seem to have been the region of the earliest and the most intensive development. In 1940 Piggott published a register of European trephined skulls known at that time (Piggott 1940: 124-127). This register gives the following areas of discovery, number of specimens and dates of discovery:

> France: 54 specimens, reported from 1876 to 1930
> Switzerland: 1 specimen, reported in 1892
> Czechoslovakia: 11 specimens, reported from 1877 to 1929
> Germany: 4 specimens, reported from 1879 to 1936
> Denmark: 7 specimens, reported from 1889 to 1938
> Sweden: 10 specimens, reported from 1913 to 1933
> Belgium: 1 specimen, reported in 1890
> Poland: 1 specimen, reported in 1916
> Portugal: 2 specimens, reported in 1880 and 1886
> Spain: 1 specimen, reported in 1919

This author gives references to published accounts and a keyed map of the sites of discovery. The large number of discoveries in France reflects not only the frequent occurence of the trait there but also the early development of archaeological interest among people of that country.

Since 1940, the date of compilation of the register above quoted, a considereable number of additional trephined specimens has been found. In 1981 Brothwell published a map indicating four cases in Ireland and one in Scotland as well as 16 in England (Brothwell 1981: 122). A considerable number of cases have probably not been reported and are now in private collections. Stewart states that "some 370 examples of the practice have been reported from the whole of prehistoric Europe, from Portugal in the southwest to Sweden in the northeast, and from England in the northwest to Czechoslovakia in the southeast" (Stewart 1958: 471). In view of the passage of time with the hazards of erosion, land exploitation and nonscientific curio gathering, the number of specimens clearly indicates a thriving practice of at least this aspect of surgery among peoples of the prehistoric past.

Where the opening of the skull is involved the mechanics of the surgery and also the post-operative care required offer exacting problems if the patient is to survive. The surgeon's task is especially difficult if his equipment is limited to non-metallic items.

The first stage in the trephining operation is the incision of the scalp which requires a very sharp knife. The blood vessels of the scalp may bleed freely and the lesion or fracture toward which the surgeon might be working might be difficult to locate. When the diploë is reached in the bone cutting, the blood flow is increased. It is accordingly important to reduce the bleeding through some sort of hemostatic measure, either physical or chemical. What the prehistoric surgeon used is conjectural, although various possibilities could have been available to him: pressure with bandaging, hemostyptic plants, soot, oil and wax. Effective methods of penetrating the skull vault were limited. One was scraping the vault area until the diploë and ultimately the inner table were penetrated, resulting in an exposure of the dura mater. Another was sawing or cutting the vault in a series of grooves or a continuous groove that eventually circumscribed a segment that could be elevated and removed. Here two options were available. Four cuts could be made, releasing a quadrilateral segment that could be lifted out. The other possibility was cutting a curvilinear groove that would ultimately release a round or oval piece of the vault.

A quite different method is possible, boring a series of holes in a circular or oval pattern and later cutting through the separating partitions and joining these in order to release a bone segment. This method was occasionally employed by the Peruvians and some other aboriginal peoples, and has come down into modern usage, but was not favored by prehistoric European surgeons, perhaps for a good reason. In this technique the operating time would have been long and with stone age equipment the cutting of the partitions between the drilled holes would have been slow and tedious (Ruffer 1918-1919: 98-99). In modern operations the use of the Gigli saw, a steel wire with sharp saw teeth, makes this method more practical. The cutting instrument used by prehistoric surgeons was undoubtedly most often a flake of igneous glasslike stone that could be chipped in order to produce a cutting or sawing edge. Oceanic peoples in historic times have used shark teeth for this purpose, but it is unlikely that early Europeans had these available. Neolithic peoples had progressed far in the technique of stone working and were able to create a blade-like implement, a saw or a pointed tool from brittle stone with great precision.

In the beginning of the operation the surgeon had to make a decision as to whether he would begin by scraping, or by cutting and sawing into the outer bone table. He might choose to thin the vault first by scraping and then proceed with a sawing maneuver, or he might begin by immediately cutting grooves. For small openings, scraping without cutting could have been satisfactory, but for large trephined areas some cutting appears to have been favored. A combination of the two was often employed. Some degree of scraping has an advantage in that the bone residue acts as a bridge for the formation of new bone.

If cutting and sawing was to be done, the surgeon had a further decision to make. Was the line of the cutting to be straight or curvilinear? There were advantages in both methods. In cutting straight lines, usually in a rectangular pattern with four cuts, the time of the operation was shorter and the task easier for the surgeon. Since a straight line cut across a curvilinear surface tends to produce a deeper cut in the high point of the curve, more damage to the dura mater of the brain was likely than with the curvilinear cut that, when carefully done, could follow the spherical form of the brain surface with less chance of penetrating the dura mater and less hazard to the patient (Parry 1936: 170). The normal four cut operation released a quadrilateral segment, whereas the curvilinear procedure released a round or oval bone segment. It has been suggested that a form of cutting compass with stone points may have been used in making the round openings (Guilard 1930: 85-86). The rectilinear sawing operation was apparently the least successful in general, not only because the dura mater was more likely to be penetrated and the brain damaged, but also because less bone debris was created that could have helped healing and bone restitution (Furstenburg 1930: 436-437; cf. MacEwen 1912: 138-145).

At the end of the operation the surgeon had further options. Was the opening to be covered with a durable plate or "stopper" made of gourd, shell, bone or metal, or left open? The purpose of the covering could have been not only to protect the trephined area from external damage, but also from the hazard of brain hemorrhage from the inside (Hrdlička 1939: 174-175). Although there was a possible chance of damage in leaving the opening without a hard covering, there were perhaps physiological advantages in so doing, since the danger of infection would have been greater and bone repair inhibited when a covering plate was inserted. Whether for the reason of physiology or convenience, the "stopper" seems usually to have been dispensed with.

It is quite possible that a number of prehistoric operations on the head were not complete perforating trephinations, but a scraping action to remove only the outer table of the skull vault and perhaps some of the diploë, but none of the inner table. An operation in recent and perhaps current use by the Bakhtiari of western Iran is of this type. Among these people the operation is performed solely in order to relieve the effects of a skull fracture that has resulted from an accident or combat. The immediate purpose of the operation is to remove the fragments of shattered bone and apply some supposedly healing medication. Healing takes place in from 20 to 30 days. Care is taken not to cut into the dura mater (Roney 1954: 489-490).

Efforts in the way of postoperative care in prehistoric times were probably few. One thing that the prehistoric patients had in their favor was a minimum of contamination and infection through close association with people and the use of uncleansed instruments and equipment from patient to patient. Communities were small and the environment unpolluted.

How successful the Neolithic trephiners were in aiding their patients, or at least in not promoting their demise, can be fairly well determined by examining the trephine wounds on skulls for evidence of healing. Survival of a patient for several weeks, or in some cases less, after the operation results in bone reaction that can be recognized as closing of the diploë and the smoothing of the rough margins of the cuts and scrapes (Lisowski 1967: 666). Piggott notes that the proportion of survivals from the operation is "extremely high." Brothwell states that "over 50 percent of the cases known show complete healing" (Brothwell 1981: 123). A fairly ample proportion of the cases that have been analyzed seem to indicate recovery, at least for a time. This leads to the conclusion that the prehistoric surgeon was quite accomplished in dealing with the intricacies invovled in this, a quite delicate operation.

The question of anesthesia during trephine and other primitive operations often arises. It is quite possible that the prehistoric surgeon had at his disposal herbs that could have lessened the pain or induced unconsciousness. Some of the narcotic plants, such as the mushroom fly-agaric employed in Siberia to produce ecstasy and the temporary derangement of the senses during the course of ceremonial frenzies, with proper dosage and administration could well have been used as medical narcotics. The Egyptians may have used opium (Lisowski 1967: 660). In some trephinations recently observed in Africa the shock seems not to have been sufficiently great to prevent the patient from walking unaided after the operation. The same was true of trephined Cornish miners in the nineteenth century (Ciba Symposia 1939: 197). What may have been used as an anesthetic, if anything, in recent African operations is a guarded secret of the medicine men although grape and palm wine could have been used to appease the suffering patient.

The motive for the operation undoubtedly determined the specific technical approach. A frequent practical reason could have been the removal of splintered bone after an injury and the elevation of depressed vault fragments that impinged on the brain coverings. Unfortunate incidents occurring in hunting and warfare involving falls, encounters with wild animals and conflicts with other humans armed with clubs or spears could well have led to such head injuries.

Trephinations appear to have been practiced most frequently in areas where weapons that could produce skull fracture were used (Ackerknecht 1968: 9). The surgeon probably had enough empirical knowledge at his disposal to realize that such areas of injury were in some way connected with the patient's distress and perhaps erratic behavior. The answer would have been to remove the depressed fragments of bone and torn flesh. In such cases a trephination would have been indicated and the surgeon accordingly would have attempted to cut out a segment of the skull that included the crushed bone. This may often have been quite difficult to locate since the area would have been bloody and bruised. Some trephine openings appear to have missed the damaged area probably for this reason. The time required to perform such an operation has been estimated on the basis of experiments to be a little more than one half hour.

The area of the skull most frequently trephined in the European specimens is the left parietal, with a second preference for the frontal bone, especially in specimens from Czechoslovakia and Denmark (Piggott 1940: 123). The frequent involvement of the left parietal area is perhaps to be explained by the likelihood that a fighting man, who would have usually been right-handed, would swing his weapon from his right side and strike his victim on the left side (Chauvet 1936: 73). If his weapon was a spear or lance the victim would be struck on the forehead. The reason for differences in the area of injury in different regions could perhaps be explained by differences in the type of weapon in prevailing use. The fact that Neolithic trephinations are usually in the parietal bone and commonly on the left side has also been attributed to the probability that a right-handed surgeon faced his patient and manipulated his instrument with his right hand (Ruffer 1918-1919: 103).

A number of the Neolithic trephined skulls are those of females and young persons, which would tend to refute the suggestion that most of the injuries were the result of military encounters. Also a number of the skulls that have been trephined show no sign of injury. The lack of traumatic indication, however, is not particularly significant since injured skulls may have had small penetrating depressed fractures all evidence of which could have been removed by the trephining operation (Ruffer 1918-1919: 97).

An unusual body of data emerged with regard to a number of skulls that were found in 1865 in central France near Paris. These had been trephined with round or oval openings. None showed pathological indications. Along with them were bone segments of varied shapes that were obviously pieces of skull vaults, presumably removed by trephination. Some had been drilled and others had a groove cut around them in the middle as though a cord had been attached in order to suspend them, presumably from the neck (Fletcher 1882: 14, also Plate I, figure 5). Other perforated items in the same dolmen included pieces of long bones and mollusc shells. These items were called amulets because of their supposed use. The round or oval fragments were termed rondelles (Fr. *rondelle* = ring or round shield). Some rondelles were not perforated. It has been suggested that these were carried in a net (Chauvet 1936: 88). Rondelles have been made the subject of complex speculations as to their meaning (Guiard 1930: 41-45).

The most plausible theory as to their possible significance was that they were thought to possess supernatural properties and were used to ward off evil forces or attract favorable influences. It was proposed that a person who recovered from a trephine operation possessed mystical properties and that a fragment of his body was able to convey some of the property to the person who wore it as an amulet. It was further suggested that the amulet was perhaps of particular value in protecting the wearer against acquiring the disease or disorder that had been the occasion for the trephine operation on the patient who had provided the rondelle.

A question also developed as to whether the rondelles were those removed from living persons who had undergone the trephine operation or had been taken shortly after the death of certain individuals. There is no valid answer to this dilemma since premortem and early post-mortem trephine markings would be indistiguishable. Both situations could have prevailed. It is the custom among the living Italian Umbrians to carry discoidal amulets prepared from fragments of human skulls as a means of preventing epilepsy (Guiard 1930: 43). A skull was found in 1938 in Crichel Down, Dorset, England, that has a circular trephine hole and the rondelle set in place. This skull had apparently been trephined during life but the patient died during or shortly after the operation (Piggott 1940: 132). The large rondelle (74.2 mm. × 65.7mm.) had been replaced and held in position during burial probably by some kind of bandage. The meaning of the find can only be guessed at with the suggestion that the rondelle was perhaps carefully kept with the skull so that no part of the deceased would be at large and subject to sympathetic magic employed to work harm toward the dead person's spirit.

The location of trephine openings with reference to the proximity of the trephine hole to the sutures in the skull has been noted with considerable interest. In general in prehistoric European trephining the sagittal suture seems to have been avoided, but there are a few notable exceptions. A skull found in Gillhog, a grave in southern Sweden of Neolithic age, had been trephined squarely in the middle of the skull on the sagittal suture between the bregma and the lambda. The opening is oblong and the margins are tapered through scraping. There is evidence of healing and the patient survived for at least three months and perhaps much longer (Persson 1976-1977: 57-59).

Another type of surgical scar found in a limited number of skulls from the Neolithic of France and some other areas is a T-shaped roughened groove that follows the sagittal suture and crosses the two parietal bones toward the back of the skull. In some cases the transverse bar of the scar forms a Y-shape rather than a T in its relation to the longitudinal bar of the scar ((Guiard 1930: 72). In most cases the groove goes through the outer table but does not penetrate the inner table. This type of scar has been called a sincipital T.*

These scars apparently were produced by cauterization with a heated stone or perhaps hot oil. Most seem to have been made during the early life of the individual (MacCurdy 1924 Vol. 2: 166). These scars are found mainly on female skulls. The very rough condition of the scar areas is apparently the result of infection, probably caused by unwashed skin or contaminated oil (Moodie 1921: 220). The burning effect of the cauterization occasionally resulted in a perforation of the inner table and a consequent "trephine by cauter-

---

*Sincipital = referring to the upper part of the cranium (derived from sin-, a variant of semi- and cipit, a variant of caput, head).

ization" (Guiard 1930: 74). Also it has been suggested that some of these scars may have been made by scraping rather than by cauterization (McKenzie 1927: 358). The geographical distribution of the sincipital T scars is limited for the most part to a region around 50 km. northwest of Paris, but some are reported from central Asia, the Canary Islands, Africa and America (Guiard 1930; Moodie 1921: 219-221).

The reason for the sincipital T operation has been debated, but the prevailing opinion is that this was done as a cure for headache, melancholia, epilepsy, and various nervous conditions that involved convulsions (Moodie 1921: 220; Sigerist 1951: 113). Their origin has also been said to be in religion, war, penal justice, mourning, therapeutics and coiffure. It has also been suggested that the T shape may have had some hieratic meaning, as a part of symbolism in a priestly cult. Also the T shape was said to be a convenience for the operator in view of the lines of parting of the hair (MacCurdy 1905: 18). It has been proposed that the predominance of female patients involved may suggest that it was used on women as a less radical therapy than the trephination that was employed on men for similar conditions (Guiard 1930: 79).

Cauterization, which was apparently the cause of the sincipital T scars, apparently continued in use from Neolithic times into the Mediaeval period as a cure for melancholia through reducing the amount of cold humors in the head (Moodie August 1920: 856). Another proposal is that prehistoric people performed the operation for hygienic purposes as was the case in New Britain where the natives trephined healthy young persons as a device for assuring a long life (Crump 1901: 168). Modern Melanesians trephine infants as a preventive against headaches in adult life (Stewart 1976: 415). Yet it must be borne in mind that some strictly ritual reasons could have applied such as initiation and exorcism rites.

Also, it is difficult to determine in many cases whether a patient died during or immediately after the operation, and whether his death was the result of the condition for which the operation was performed, or was caused by the operation itself. Some trephine operations may have been performed on skulls at some time after the patients' death. This could have been for the practical purpose of training surgeons in the technique of the operation. Also, there is the possibility that it may have been thought that a piece of the skull of a deceased person preserved some of the mystical power and spiritual property of the individual when he was alive, in the manner of a religious relic (Wakefield and Dellinger 1939: 167).

The prehistoric surgeon was not a scientific practitioner and, while he often possessed a considerable degree of skill and some empirical knowledge of operative and healing procedures, the culture in which he worked was without doubt highly charged with mysticism and fostered practices aimed at the appeasement of supernatural forces. Regardless of his own intellectual approach to his professional activities, he probably carried out his ministrations in an atmosphere of supernatural precepts and his healing efforts had to harmonize with the cultural matrix of his society.

Operations on the skull were the prime surgical achievement of prehistoric surgeons as far as archaeologically recovered evidence indicates. Yet much other surgery may have been practiced since it is unlikely that the skill and design inolved in trephining would not have been paralleled in some other surgical activities. While specific evidence of these areas is lacking, or uncertain, two types of surgical operation may be cited as probable.

Amputation of arms, legs and fingers or toes would have been likely. A hunter could have suffered from a mangled arm or leg through the violent attack of a wild animal. A person pinned under a rockfall could have been seriously maimed. In such cases the removal of the lacerated member would have seemed necessary for the survival of the individual. The same could have been true of frostbitten hands and feet with subsequent degeneration of tissue. The technique of managing both bone and skin in an amputation would probably not have been difficult for people who were accustomed to skin and butcher large wild animals for food purposes and to prepare and work pelts. A problem would have been to arrest the flow of blood from severed arteries and manage the skin flaps for a satisfactory covering. The loss of blood could have been arrested through pressure and bandaging with perhaps some use of hemostatic applications. The manipulations and suturing of skin flaps was probably well within the scope of people accustomed to skin animals and cut and sew hides in the making of pouches, bags and clothing. Sinews for suturing could have been prepared in same way as those used in the finishing and hafting of weapons.

A different aspect of amputation is indicated in the wall paintings in some prehistoric caves.

In Gargas Cave, a prehistoric cave in southern France, a number of human hands have been stenciled on the walls. These had apparently been made by holding the left hand flat against the cave wall and then dusting the pigment with the right hand or blowing the pigment in order to outline the hand form on the wall (Moodie 1920(d): 1301). A number of these show missing fingers, some representing the hand as a series of stump digits. There are three possible explanations. Perhaps certain fingers were doubled under as the pigment was applied; a mutilating disease, such as leprosy, had destroyed the fingers; or the fingers had been amputated before the stencils were made. Bending the fingers under sufficiently to make the stencil show the fingers as defined stumps would have been anatomically difficult; and there is no evidence of mutilating bone disease in bones of comparable antiquity (leprosy did not occur in Europe until Mediaeval times [Steinbock 1976: 194-195]). This leaves the most plausible explanation to be the amputation of fingers before the stencils were made (Macalister 1921: 458). This well could have been for certain cultural reasons such as mourning, punishment or initiation rites (Brothwell 1967: 68). There is a possibility that the loss of fingers may have been the result of frostbite, but stenciled hands on the cave walls of Castillo and Font-de-Gome, where similar exposure to freezing weather probably prevailed, do not show the indications of missing digits (Macalister 1921: 458).

Ancient Stone Age surgery continued into later cultures in certain of its techniques. Trephining the skull was practiced in Greek, Roman and Mediaeval times and into the present. Methods used in ancient times were not mechanically much different from those employed in more recent surgery except that metal technology made possible the use of more refined and efficient instruments. The reasons for performing the operation have changed progressively with increasing physiological understanding of the brain and pathological conditions associated with it. Cauterization continued into the Middle Ages and later as a means of arresting excessive blood flow and preventing infection. There is little knowledge available concerning amputation practices of ancient peoples although the amputation of fingers, for whatever reason, seems to have been sometimes done. Manipulative surgery in the form of fracture reduction and the reduction of dislocations has left no authentic indication from the prehistoric past since some of these conditions can be cured by nature without human intervention. Well healed fractures without serious misalignment have been found in the bones of wild anthropoid apes and presumably could have occurred at times in prehistoriuc humans without artificial assistance (Schultz 1967: 53).

Neolithic man as a patient probably approached the treatment of his illnesses in somewhat the same way that we do today. A minor illness, such as a common cold or sore throat, was no doubt treated through household measures: heat applied by means of pressed leaves or a warmed stone and possibly herb extracts that had been found by experience to be beneficial. In the same attitude that, when harassed by more serious involvements such as headache, back pains, nausea or confusion and weakness, we have recourse to physicians or unconventional therapists, the sufferer of the Stone Age probably appealed to the healing professionals of his culture: shamans or witch doctors. Some of these had a degree of empirical knowledge and skill. These may have included practitioners of several grades. The less elite probably did little more than lance boils and extract teeth, all with a boast of competence and a flourish of ceremonialism. Others would have been experts, more or less, in trephination and amputation. There is ample reason to believe that the elite of these ancient doctors were in considerable degree trained and profited by a fund of more or less institutionalized experience. Some no doubt were bunglers who performed their operations with high claims and mysterious embellishment but disastrously crude technique. Whatever doctrinal base there may have been for prehistoric surgery is unknown, but the skill and precision involved in some of the operations and the survival of the patients gives clear evidence that certain of the ancient practitioners were technically qualified for their undertakings.

In general prehistoric surgery demonstrates progress in surgical skills to an impressive level of technical ability considering Stone Age instrumentation. At the same time the doctrinal and theoretical base for ancient practices was perhaps fantastic, mainly supernatural and certainly prescientific. Yet the patient may often have been aided by the surgeon's ministrations. A combination of technical skill, some degree of empirical knowledge, traditional authority and a high degree of confidence on the part of the patient in the surgeon's ability could well have brought about a successful healing in many cases of injury and illness.

CHAPTER 2

CLASSICAL ANTIQUITY

Egypt, Greece, Rome and India

Surgical Knowledge of the Egyptians

THE NILE VALLEY is a unique part of the world and has a
history that results from its geography. As a fertile strip ten to
fourteen miles wide running north and south in north Africa for
over 500 miles it has had contacts to the north with the Mediterranean and the world of the Greeks and Romans, and to the south
with the cultures of Black Africa. It developed independently a
dynamic cultural force that was unique and gradually inserted itself
into the civilizations of Europe. A strange dualism emerged in Egyptian culture. On the one side was an extremely practical
workmanlike dedication to purpose in creating enormous structures
of stone in accord with canons of design that have been among the
world's greatest aesthetic achievements.

On the other hand Egyptian culture was saturated with a concern
for mystic forces that were symbolized in birds, mammals and rep-
tiles, and in esoteric emblems. The Egyptians recognized the primal
forces of sun, sky, air and water as the source of life and human
energy. The sun was shown as a falcon-headed man who wore the sun
disk as a crown. The sky was considered the mother of the sun and
stars and was represented as a cow and at times as a woman. The
forces of cosmic order had their relationship to humans, their problems and stresses. The spiritual progress of the individual human

was traced into an afterlife with the weighing by Osiris of his soul against a feather in determining the judgment of the individual.

Medicine in Egypt reflected this dualism in doctrine. One aspect was practical and naturalistic; the other was mystical, hyperphysical and folkloristic. Accidents or conflicts that involved contusions and fractures were regarded as mundane events and these called for naturalistic investigation and treatment. Diseases and systemic disorders, on the other hand, were believed to be caused by antagonistic spirits, and against these only the powers of magic could be effective. The two approaches to healing were often confused. The roles of physician and priest were frequently combined.

In practical matters such as architecture, geometry and astronomy, the Egyptians generated a progressive, logical and aesthetically sensitive pattern of culture. On the other hand their mythology and religion were obscure, fantastic and incomprehensible, perhaps having been derived in some measure from the aboriginal folk religions of the sub-Saharan populations to the south. Max Müller refers to "the unintelligibility of the Egyptian religion, which in its hyperconservatism, absolutely refused to be adapted to reason" (Max Müller 1918: 7). In this matrix of polytheistic mysticism the medical concepts of the Egyptians emerged, using some measures of practical therapy but also at times abounding in magic, references to the deities and mysteriously compounded medications. Much of the detail of Egyptian medical practices is unknown, but a few surviving documents have preserved the major aspects for certain historical periods.

The natural conditions in Egypt for the preservation of antiquities have been favorable because of the warm, dry climate of much of the Nile Valley. In addition Egyptian culture fostered beliefs that required, for a portion of their populace, the preservation of human bodies and assemblages of artifacts in well sealed burial sites. On the adverse side the technical refinements, aesthetic fascination and intrinsic value of Egyptian artifacts have brought about the looting and destruction of archaeological sites almost from the time that they were supposedly closed for eternity. Some knowledge of Egyptian surgery has been gained through the study of mummified and entombed bodies, but the most extensive source of data is in the interpretation of a few papyri, documents inscribed on reed paper, that were intentionally shielded from destructive forces and have ultimately reached modern experts for decipherment.

The main ancient Egyptian documents that throw some light on medicine are the Ebers papyrus, the Edwin Smith papyrus, the Hearst papyrus, the Chester Beatty papyrus and the Kahun papyrus. The Ebers papyrus is the longest and is mainly concerned with the naming of ailments without diagnostic description, and recipes for treatment interspersed with magical spells and incantations. The Hearst papyrus is of later date and is apparently based on the same sources as Ebers papyrus. The Chester Beatty papyrus is primarily devoted to diseases of the anus and rectum, and may be considered a treatise on proctology interlarded with magic and spells. The Kahun papyrus is ancient but fragmentary and is concerned with one area only, gynecology.

The document that throws the most light on surgical procedures is the Edwin Smith papyrus. Before discussing the information in regard to surgery conveyed by the Edwin Smith papyrus it is important to give brief consideration to the nature of Egyptian magic since it seems to have been part of all medical practice, even the most matter of fact surgical manipulations. Names of divinities were used in prayers of appeal, but also the names themselves were often thought to have mystical power. At times the names of ancient gods no longer worshipped and largely forgotten were used as conjuring devices. Mystic numbers were often conjured with and prescribed numerical repetitions were involved in the healing formulas. The following spell for the removal of a bone stuck in a person's throat is typical of a magical approach that was perhaps combined with a minor surgical manipulation.

SPELL FOR REMOVING A BONE FROM THE THROAT

I am he whose head reacheth the sky,
And whose feet reach the abyss,
Who hath awakened the crocodile of wax in Pe-zeme of Thebes;
For I am So, Sime, Tamaho,
This is my correct name.
Anuk, Anuk!
For a hawk's egg is what is in my mouth,
An ibis's egg is what is in my belly.
Therefore, bone of god,

Bone of man,
Bone of bird,
Bone of fish,
Bone of animal,
Bone of anything,
None being excepted;
Therefore, that which is in thy belly,
Let it come to thy chest!
That which is in thy chest,
Let it come to thy mouth!
That which is in thy mouth,
Let it come to my hand now!
For I am he who is in the seven heavens,
Who standeth in the seven sanctuaries,
For I am the son of the living god.

This is to be repeated seven times over a cup of water which is then to be given to the patient to drink and after that (with perhaps some assistance by the physician) the bone was supposed to emerge. It will be noted that the name of a divinity is important and the number seven is a part of the spoken incantation as well as the number of times it is to be repeated. A physician working in this style of practice must have memorized a considerable number of spells along with the details of their application and perhaps in addition may have had some recourse to folk medications and minor surgical techniques.

The Edwin Smith papyrus is named for an antiquarian who was perhaps the first American to devote himself to a thorough investigation of Egyptian inscriptions and artifacts. He studied Egyptian cultures in London, Paris and Cairo and in 1862 acquired in Luxor the papyrus scroll with which his name is associated. On his death in 1906 his daughter gave it to the New York Historical Society and later it was entrusted to James Henry Breasted of the University of Chicago for translation and interpretation. His findings were published in detail in 1930 (Breasted 1930). This manuscript is a roll slightly over fifteen feet long, written on both sides and including nearly 500 lines of hieratic Egyptian script. It deals with 48 cases of clinical surgery arranged in logical sequence from the head downward, beginning with gashes and fractures of the skull such as those that could have been produced by blows with a sword, and including injuries to the jaw, neck and collarbone, and finally the lower spinal column. At this point the text comes to an abrupt end, suggesting that it had been copied from an older document and that the remainder was either lost or disregarded. It was written about 1600 B.C. and was presumably a copy of a manuscript written about 3000 B.C. There are explanatory notes or glosses that interpret certain unusual or obsolete expressions. These are in the language of the Middle Kingdom, 2080-1640 B.C.

Breasted refers to the Edwin Smith papyrus as the "oldest body of science now extant" (Breasted 1930: 43). The essence of the document is a series of case descriptions and analyses, along with clinical directions. Each resume consists of the following:

1. Title: The designation of the injury and the location of the organ or place in the body affected.
2. Examination: This involves instruction to a second person, perhaps a learner, as to how he should examine the patient, e.g. where he should look, feel, probe, etc.
3. Diagnosis: This always begins, "Thou shouldst say concerning him . . ." followed by a brief identification of the patient's condition and ending with one of the three comments, "An ailment which I shall treat; an ailment with which I will contend; or an ailment not to be treated."
4. Treatment: This instruction is usually far from detailed but does commonly refer to closing wounds, bandaging, perhaps stitching and cauterizing, binding with fresh meat, or doing nothing.

The following is an example of a case that involves a flesh wound on the head above the eyebrow, but not a bone fracture. (Case No. 10 in Breasted's sequence. The original manuscript had no numerical designations. Breasted 1930: 225-233.)

"Instructions concerning a wound in the top of his eyebrow: If you examine a man having a wound in the top of his eyebrow, penetrating to the bone, you should palpate his wound and draw his gash together for him with stitching. You should say concerning him: 'He has a wound in his eyebrow, an ailment which I shall treat.' Now after you have stitched it, you should bind fresh meat upon it the first day. If you find that the stitching of his wound is loose, you should draw it together for him with two strips and you should treat it with grease and honey every day until he recovers" (Breasted 1930: 226-233).

The strips referred to here are probably of linen soaked in sticky resin. The stitching indicated is probably a continuous suture as used in a few of the late Egyptian mummies after removing the internal viscera (Breasted 1930: 8). It has been proposed, however, that the characters used for "stitching" may have meant some form of clamp (Sigerist 1951: 345).

Case No. 4 involves "a gaping wound in the head penetrating to the bone and splitting the skull; an ailment with which I will contend." The attendant learner or assistant is told to palpate the wound and if the patient shudders exceedingly and discharges blood from his nostrils and ears, and is unable to look at his two shoulders and his breast . . . (unfortunately the remainder of the diagnosis is lost). By way of treatment the patient is supported with bricks (supposedly in order to restrict movement of his head), and grease is to be applied to his head. Thereafter he is apparently left to the healing power of nature. In one case (No. 6) a wound of the skull is described where the brain surface is exposed, but this is classed as "an ailment that cannot be treated." Not all the cases where the condition is dismissed as untreatable are consigned to immanent death, however, since even with the "untreatable" designation some cases involve directions for nursing and care.

Case No. 36 involves a fracture of the humerus. The description and healing instructions for treatment read: "If thou examinist a man having a break in his upper arm and findest his upper arm hanging down, separated from its fellow, an ailment which I shall treat, thou shouldest place him prostrate on his back, with something folded between his two shoulder blades; thou shouldest spread out with his two shoulders in order to stretch apart his upper arm until that break falls in place. Thou shouldest make for him two splints of linen, and thou shouldest apply for him one of them both on the inside of his arm, and the other of them both on the under side of his arm. Thou shouldest bind it with *ymrw* [an unidentified mineral] and treat afterward with honey every day until he recovers" (Breasted 1930: 354-357).

The means of applying traction here are not clear, but the phrase "falls into place" would seem to imply that a good apposition of the bone fragments is expected. Splints "of linen" were probably wooden slats wrapped with linen bandages. The surgeon's apparently assured approach to the case would seem to indicate that such fractures were a common occurrence in his practice.

Several types of dislocation are noted. Instructions for reducing a dislocated jaw include the direction, "you should put your thumbs upon the ends of the two rami of the mandible in the inside of his mouth and your fingers under his chin, and you should cause them to fall back so that they rest in their places." This for many centuries has been a standard technique. Dislocations and fractures were probably quite frequent among the Egyptian workers since there must have been fairly frequent falls from high scaffolds made of frail materials used in the construction of tall buildings and monuments. In one case (No. 33) a fracture of the cervical vertebrae is attributed to "his falling headlong" and being struck on his head, driving the vertebrae of his neck into the next, creating an impacted fracture (Breasted 1930: 338). This was classed as "an ailment not to be treated." An examination of over 5,000 skeletons recovered from one series of excavations revealed that 3 percent had fractures apparently having resulted from accident, warfare or perhaps beating (Breasted 1930: 11; Sigerist 1951: 345).

Bandaging with fresh flesh is frequently noted, perhaps as a means of stopping the bleeding of a wound. There is no mention of any cutting or debridement of wounds, although probable suturing and the use of adhesive strips is cited in several cases. Various medications are referred to as salve for wounds. All the ingredients are not known, although honey was a frequent component. Cauterization is referred to in one case for the treatment of an abscess-like tumor. The condition is indicated as "an ailment which I shall treat with a fire-drill."

This is an interesting reference since it is one of the very few instances where a specific surgical instrument is cited. The reference is apparently to cauterization in which the fire-drill, a device usually used in creating fires for domestic and other uses, is employed to generate the heat needed for surgical cauterization. The frictional heat created by twirling the shaft between the palms of the hands was great enough to ignite a fire where the end of the shaft rotated in the socket of the hearth plate, and the shaft itself could have been used as a cauterizing implement (Harrison 1954: 222-223; Breasted 1930: 365).

There is no documentary reference to surgical instruments other than to the fire-drill mentioned above. No knife is mentioned in the Edwin Smith papyrus, yet there were probably knives of various types, forceps, probes, awls, needles and perhaps many other items in the equipment of the physician. Instruments would have been made of copper or bronze. Bronze became common in Egypt by around 2000 B.C., while iron was scarcely known until around 670 B.C. (Forbes 1954: 588, 597). On the wall of the temple at Kom Ombo an array of implements is represented on a carved stone panel. From their appearance these items appear to be surgical instruments, although their identity as such has been questioned (Sigerist 1951: 346).

Singer and Underwood, on the other hand, illustrate this panel, stating the date to be around 100 B.C. and identify the various instruments as a probe director, forceps, saws, a retractor, cauteries, shears, a sponge and scalpels (Singer and Underwood 1962: 9). This identification would seem to be correct through comparison of the form of these implements with later known surgical equipment such as that from Pompeii. Also it would seem unlikely that craftsman's tools would be illustrated in carvings on a sanctified temple wall. There would have been a logical reason for displaying the accouterments of the surgeon, since physicians had both a medical and a priestly role in their professional activities.

Singer and Underwood feel that the instruments represented are typical of those in earlier use in Egypt. The Egyptians used a variety of splints in dealing with fractures. These were often made of bark and palm fiber in the form of a tube, and would have had no effect in restoring the alignment of displaced bone fragments. Shortening of limbs and misalignment of broken bones would have been inevitable (Moodie 1920(b): 352-357). The papyrus Hearst mentions a bandage covered with flour made from beans, barley, cream and honey. On drying this could have had the effect of a plaster cast (Sigerist 1951: 344).

The Edwin Smith papyrus mentions two types of splint. One was of wood probably lined with linen, two of which were bound to a fractured arm or leg. These are referred to in the text as being "of linen," and Breasted suggests that they might possibly have been of cloth, stiffened with plaster or gum, forming a type of cast (Breasted 1930: 190). The other type of splint mentioned was a roll of linen forming a more or less solid post and used in treating a broken nose or a dislocated clavicle.

G. Elliot Smith describes two cases of the application of splints to broken bones found at Naga-ed-eder, about 100 miles north of Luxor, and dating back to the Fifth Dynasty around 2500 B.C. to 2350 B.C. One instance is a compound fracture of the shaft of the right femur of a fourteen-year-old girl. Four splints were applied, each consisting of a strip of roughly surfaced wood wrapped in a linen bandage. The largest splint is 40.3 cm. long, 32 mm. wide and 7 mm. thick. The splints were held in place by a linen bandage. They would have had no value in preventing a shortening of the limb and displacement of bone fragments. The other case involved a compound fracture of the left forearm. In this instance the splint consisted of a tube of three pieces of rough bark and a bundle of straws of coarse grass, all wrapped in linen. These two are probably the oldest splints of which there is any record and splints of the same type have been in use in Egypt into recent times (Smith 1908: 732-733).

Trephining the skull was apparently not practiced in Egypt, certainly not to any great extent. One case, however, has been noted, that of a person of a noble family of the Twelfth Dynasty, between 2000 B.C. and 1788 B.C. It was found at Lisht, where the ruined pyramid of Amenemhet is located (Breasted 1930: 596).

It is possible that the Egyptians may have been capable in the area of amputations. There are pictorial representations at Thebes and Dendara of amputated limbs, and excavations at the pyramid of Medum have revealed that one man lost his left leg and that another had his hand cut off and placed in the tomb. There may be some indication that the Egyptians performed lithotomies and cataract operations (Baas 1971: 18-19). Apparently all Egyptian men were circumcised (Smith 1908: 732). The practice may have involved a degree of respect for the flint knife (Berdoe 1893: 71). Castration was apparently performed frequently and efficiently since the Romans used Egypt as a source of eunuchs (Baas 1971: 18).

Dental surgery seems to have been quite rare among the Egyptians, although one case of apparent significance has been found. This was a mandible excavated at Giza in which there were two holes bored, apparently in order to drain an abscess below the first molar on the right side. Each hole is round, 2.5 mm. in diameter. The holes were placed with skill in order not to impinge on the roots of the teeth (Hooton 1917: 29-32). This specimen dates from around 1500 B.C., and is probably the oldest example of oral surgery on record.

Dental caries seem to have been rare in ancient Egypt, although attrition of the teeth was quite common, particularly among the poorer class because of the coarse food eaten. This often led to exposure of the pulp cavity and septic infection. Caries increased during the Pyramid age among the wealthier members of the population as more refined foods were included in the diet (Dawson 1964: 64).

The back side of the Edwin Smith papyrus is of later origin than the obverse and contains invocations against pestilential winds, formulas for the rejuvenation of the aged and other mystical prescriptions typical of a later historic period than that of the primary inscription. Obviously two types of medical doctrine are involved in the manuscript. An earlier ancestral treatise involves little magic, was largely naturalistic and provided a practical guide for the physician in dealing with his patients. The later document is supernatural in emphasis and mainly embodies mystical incantations where the healer was more of a priest than a physician. A shift in the orientation of the medical profession with time from the matter of fact to the supernatural is apparently indicated, although it must be borne in mind that during the later historic time when the Edwin Smith papyrus was inscribed there must have been sufficient interest in the older document to have it copied.

An important element in the character of Egyptian medicine was its rigorous adherence to tradition. There was little room for individual initiative since any deviation from the prescribed techniques would have been regarded as a violation of professional ethics and religious dogma. Therefore within each historic period the progress of surgery, and medicine in general, was advanced but little, and during the later epochs seems to have become degraded through increased emphasis on the supernatural.

An indirect contribution of Egypt to medicine and surgery may have been through the practice of mummification. Embalmers were skilled in opening the body and removing the viscera, with the exception of the heart and its appendages, which were carefully left *in situ* (Dawson 1927: 43). They were also experts in bandaging and in this capacity were called upon by physicians for surgical bandages. There was a good opportunity to learn anatomy through the embalming procedures and there seems to have been some use of it in surgery (Dawson 1967). The opening of the body cavities in the preparation of mummies did perhaps pave the way toward surgical dissection by allaying fears and avoidances in regard to molesting a dead body.

An aspect of Egyptian medicine, including surgery, was undoubtedly the powerful suggestion involved in the curative measures. While their incantations seem to us to be no more than senseless gibberish, they were probably to the suffering Egyptian patient an avenue to the cosmic powers and the favors of the gods. Whether the patient suffered from a severe headache or a violent sword cut on his skull, he would have been in some measure aided by the conviction that the arcane mysteries were being tapped in his behalf. The surgeon, while bandaging a severe wound on a patient's head, may have uttered some cabalistic pronouncements that conveyed to the sufferer the feeling that he was under the care of an agent of the gods. This certainly would have relieved his tensions and fears and could have given a better opportunity for the healing powers of nature to work in his behalf.

Early Medicine in Greece and Rome

The early development of surgery in Greece is difficult to reconstruct since there are no medical documents as such before the time of Hippocrates in the fourth century B.C. Our only literary resources are in the few references to surgical manipulations in Greek epic poetry and the retrospective interpretation of later documents that were based on the status of the art in their own time.

The beginning of Greek scientific medicine, which was the beginning of modern science in the medical realm, was in the life and the attributed work of Hippocrates (c. 460-c. 370 B.C.). The known biography of Hippocrates is minimal, but his effect on history has been tremendous. It is known that he was a physician of wide reputation, was a benevolent individual in using his knowledge for the relief of suffering mankind, that he travelled much, that he lived to an advanced age and that he was apparently the key figure in the personnel of the medical school on the island of Cos, the second largest of the Dodecanese Islands of the eastern Mediterranean off the western shore of Turkey.

He is given credit for assembling the series of over sixty books that are called the Hippocratic collection or corpus, a few, or none of which he may have authored. These documents, which may have formed a part of the library of the medical school, obviously were not all written by the same individual since they are somewhat different in style and in some respects are contradictory in content. They do, however, give us a remarkably vivid account of the status of medicine during the fourth century B.C. and mark the transition between earlier primitive folk medicine and systematic scientific methods based on careful observation, accurate recording and the analysis of human experience in the course of trauma and disease.

The findings reported in the Hippocratic corpus could not have sprung full-blown from the minds and experience of a few Coan doctors around 400 B.C. There must have been centuries of observation and practice, although undocumented, behind their summations reported in the Hippocratic records. Therefore we can refer to the Hippocratic methods as an upper limit from which we can reconstruct the surgical technology and instrumentation of the earlier period that is our concern in this discussion.

Homeric Surgery: Battlefield Methods. The insular and peninsular geography, that was the homeland of the Greek peoples and their neighbors, led to the emergence of independent city states rather than to the formation of a unified political body. This in turn promoted a continuing history of conflicts between neighbors resulting from their competitive struggle for supremacy. Added to this was the vulnerability of these peoples to attack by the waterborne forces of other peoples who had access to the Mediterranean. The result was an almost uninterrupted series of larger and smaller violent conflicts.

It is then by no means surprising that what information we have about early Greek surgery deals with the treatment of military casualties. Since the rising literary genius of the Greeks encouraged the composition and recording of traditional epic poems, and since some of these have been quite well preserved, we can consult these works for suggestions as to the early surgical and medical procedures. The Iliad of Homer, which was written in the eighth century B.C., contains over one hundred passages that mention wounds caused by arrows, javelines and hurled rocks. Wounds mentioned in the Iliad, along with their severity, are as follows:

106 spear wounds with 80% mortality
17 sword thrusts with 100% mortality
12 arrow wounds with 42% mortality

This would seem to imply that the surgeon's primary area of usefulness would have been in the treatment of arrow wounds, with occasional success in dealing with spear injuries, and that sword thrusts were beyond his capability.

An example of a Trojan War episode recorded by Homer in the Iliad is as follows:

The warrior Eurypylus was wounded and his plight was dealt with in this way:

> The attendant . . . spread the ox hide couch: then as he lay reclined, Patroclus with his dagger, from the thigh cut out the biting shaft; and from the wound with tepid water cleansed the clotted blood; then pounded in his hands a root applied, astringent, anodyne, which all his pain allayed; the wound was dried, and staunched the blood (Iliad Book 11, lines 958-967).

This was obviously an emergency operation where the only surgical instrument was a dagger. Yet some effort was made to stop the flow of blood, to cleanse the wound and to ease the patient.

Homer cites a number of war wounds produced by piercing and thrusting weapons which were treated by removing the point, if embedded in the flesh, and by bandaging, which was apparently done with considerable efficiency.

We are compelled to look in two directions for suggestions as to what the basic features of pre-Hippocratic surgery of ancient Greece were like. On the one side we have the crude battlefield methods of the professional soldier acting on occasion as an amateur surgeon in attempting to care for the injuries of his comrades, as described in the Homeric accounts. His efforts involved mainly the digging out of weapon points with his most available instrument, his dagger, or perhaps on occasion a hunting knife, after which the wound was bandaged. If the patient was an elite hero, means were probably taken to relieve the pain of his injury through some kind of soothing medication, after which he was provided with rest and relaxation.

On the other side, working backward from the status of the art represented in the Hippocratic corpus, we can note some of the outstanding Hippocratic techniques that were the probable derivatives, with improvement and amplification, of the methods that were applied during earlier centuries. Since surgery is essentially a manual art and its efficiency depends on what can be done with the hands and the extension of the hands in the form of instruments, our most useful approach is to review the range and type of instruments mentioned in the Hippocratic documents with indications as to their uses. We can, with some reason, assume that elements of this technology were in existence for several prior centuries.

Greek culture prior to Hippocrates was in a transitional phase between the Bronze age and the Iron age. This was reflected in the making of surgical instruments. An important quality in surgical devices is the sharpness of cutting blades. Particularly during the long portion of medical history before the development of anaesthetics, speed was an essential element in operations since prolonged cutting meant loss of blood and subsequent hazard to the survival of the patient. Therefore, the faster the surgeon could work the better chances his patient had for continued life. Hence the desire for sharp, smooth cutting blades was urgently felt. During the Stone Age a blade of chipped stone, often volcanic glass, was used, which gave for a time at least a sharp cutting edge, but at the best it was somewhat irregular and dulled quickly. Accordingly with the coming of metal technology bronze and iron were chosen for instrument making.

Bronze was resistive to corrosion but was not capable of maintaining a good working edge. Iron was a superior material for knives and other cutting implements. An important aspect of early iron working was that the most convenient source of heat for smelting was charcoal (Milne 1907: 12). This added carbon to the product which in effect produced an early form of steel, harder and more durable than iron. This was undoubtedly chosen for the working edges of many surgical instruments. The unfortunate feature for us, however, is that iron and steel do not survive well the deteriorating effects of time, particularly in a semi-maritime environment such as the Grecian islands. As a result our recovered arrays of surgical instruments from the early period are few and the items that have survived are mostly of bronze, whereas iron instruments, that were probably more favored by the early surgeons, have disappeared with the decomposition of time.

The surgeon's most fundamental instrument was his knife. The same knife that skinned animals, cut up meat from hunted carcasses and at times served as a weapon of offense or defense, also could have been used as a surgical device in removing embedded weapon points and opening abscesses. Knives among the early Greeks appear to have been of several forms. Hippocrates refers to a bellied scalpel which presumably had a short, wide blade that provided an efficient cutting edge for tissue operations. Also a long bladed and pointed knife is mentioned. This could have been used for opening abscesses and the debridement of wounds. The Hippocratic author also cites an implement used in bleeding, the *phlebotome*. There is no precise description of this but is was presumably a small, narrow-pointed lance or knife that could have been used for opening blood vessels and perhaps had other applications. A knife of this type would undoubtedly have been in use before Hippocrates' time since bleeding seems to have been a therapeutic resource of long standing.

Probes or sounds are also alluded to in the Hippocratic writings. These appear to have been made of metal, either bronze or tin. They were probably blunt or bulb shaped at the end and were used for exploring the various channels and passages of the body with minimal damage to tissue. There is also allusion to an ophthalmic probe although the description is not clear. There is specific reference to a probe of tin with an opening at the end similar to the eye of a large needle. A piece of lint was passed through the eye and it was used in clearing and treating fistulas and passages of the body.

The Hippocratic accounts refer to several types of uterine dilators. These were made of wood, and were of graduated sizes being inserted for examination and subsequent treatment. They are described as being made of smooth pine wood, round and having the shape of the index finger. Six were used. There is also mention of dilators made of lead or tin and fitted with wooden handles.

Bleeding cups were probably in use from very early times in Greece as well as elsewhere. The earliest ones were probably of horn and later ones were made of ceramic material, glass or metal. The earlier usage was probably to suck on the horn through an opening at the tip in order to reduce the atmospheric pressure within the cup. In later practice the cup was heated with a smoldering substance before being applied to the patient's body. As it cooled atmospheric pressure within the cup decreased, creating suction and furthering the extravasation of blood. Hippocrates mentions bronze cups with no openings that were apparently used in this way.

The use of enemas was apparently common in earlier and later Greek medicine. The earlier syringes consisted of a tube, perhaps of metal or reed, to which was attached the bladder of an animal or a bag formed from animal skin. Hippocrates mentions both rectal and vaginal injections with this type of apparatus and also the use of a blacksmith's bellows in order to dilate the intestine before giving an enema in treating intestinal constrictions.

Cauterization was quite common in Hippocratic medicine and no doubt much earlier. The Hippocratic accounts refer to several types of cauteries, spoken of as "irons," indicating that this was the usual material of which they were made. They were perhaps occasionally made of bronze, but this was less desirable since this material softens and does not hold heat as well as iron. Cauteries were used for a number of purposes: arresting the flow of blood, the removal of tumors, and as counterirritants. Some were referred to as nail shaped, which probably indicated a thin quadrangular form, and others with ends in the shape of a coin.*

---

*With time, cauterizing irons took on a fantastic variety of forms. Costaeus writing on caustics in A.D. 1595 describes these forms as "thin and thick, sharp and dull." He describes some as shaped like a date seed, others lentil shaped, some like the head of a water lily, some resembling a sword, some shaped like the Greek letter gamma, some like a sharp stylus, some round, some quadrate and others of various invented forms (Costaeus 1595: 43). It is quite likely that the pre-Hippocratic surgeon may have expressed considerable ingenuity in devising these.

The Hippocratic accounts mention raspatories or bone scrapers which were applied to broken bones and fragments after fractures. There are no surviving early examples of these from the Hippocratic period but they were probably quite similar to the modern periosteal raspatory.

There is some confusion in the Hippocratic documents in regard to the identification of saws and trephines. A saw is mentioned several times but the context would indicate that the reference is to a type of trephine, since circular motion is described. The Greek word used is the term applied to saws such as those employed in cutting stone, but Hippocrates apparently referred to an instrument somewhat like the trephine of more recent times, a metallic cylinder with saw teeth cut in the perimeter at one end (Phillips 1973: 105). It may be assumed that the Hippocratics used a circular trephine for the removal of bone fragments from a skull that had suffered a depressed fracture.

To what degree we may imply that a form of circular trephine was used earlier is open to question, since the precise cutting of saw teeth in a tube of iron or steel is a difficult technical procedure. Trephining by scraping or by cutting linear grooves in a quadrangular form or perhaps by drilling holes in a circle and cutting through the separations would have been possible techniques prior to more advanced metal fabrication. It is a reasonable conclusion that the circular trephine was not in the array of surgical equipment until late in pre-Hippocratic times.

The Hippocratic accounts mention an elevator used in raising the protruding or sunken portions of a fractured bone. There is no indication of what this was like, but it most probably was a form of levering instrument similar to the "Lane elevator" of recent manufacture.

In dealing with cases where childbirth was difficult and normal labor appeared impossible, Hippocrates advised breaking up the head and removing the fetal body with bone forceps and a traction hook. Traction hooks of later origin have survived, and the earlier ones were probably more or less the same, being a semicircular hook that could have been used to withdraw the dead or partially destroyed fetus. Those of early origin were probably quite similar to the modern obstetrical crotchet.

It is quite possible that the Hippocratic surgeon, and also the pre-Hippocratic surgeon, had some form of uterine curette. This may have been no more than a form of the strigil, the scraper used on the bodies of athletes after violent exercise (Milne 1907: 157).

From this review of Hippocratic surgical instruments and their presumed uses, we are able to cite a few tentative indications.

The pre-Hippocratic surgeon, somewhat after the end of the Trojan War around 1000 B.C., could have had in his operating kit the following:

- Several types of knives, at least one with a long and pointed blade, and another with a short, wide blade.
- Probes or sounds, some with an eye opening for the insertion of a linen strip for cleansing tubes and channels.
- Uterine dilators of graduated sizes, made of wood.
- Bleeding cups, some of horn, others perhaps of pottery or bronze.
- Enema syringes, made of a hollow tube to which was attached the bladder of an animal or a skin sack.
- Cauterizing irons of several shapes.
- Raspatories for scraping bone.
- An elevator for lifting fractured pieces of bone.
- Perhaps a traction hook or crotchet to assist in the removal of a dead fetus.

Other items were most probably included, which would have been forceps of several shapes, shears and sewing needles, some undoubtedly of the three cornered type the sharp corners of which would have aided in passing the needle through firm human skin. The surgeon would also have had available strips of linen for bandages, various medications, some of which were probably hemostatic, and others anaesthetic.

Primitive forms of the instruments above mentioned would have been replaced by more refined designs during Hippocratic times, and still further improved and supplemented by the time of Galen during the second century A.D.

In general the Greek surgeon a century before Hippocrates probably had a range of instrumental equipment which, although crude, could have been capable of many basic surgical maneuvers. The forms of many of his instruments may have been elementary as compared with Hippocratic and later Roman designs, but with what was available in the way of instruments together with his knowledge, transmitted to him by word of mouth from an earlier generation of doctors, he was no doubt able to relieve much of the suffering of his patients.

Early Roman surgical practice is not well documented but was in all probability much the same as that of Greece. Numerous Greek physicians were brought to Rome, many as slaves, and the more advanced methods of the Greeks accordingly became a part of Roman medical technology. The only Roman writer who has given us much information in regard to medicine in general and surgery in particular is Aurelius Cornelius Celsus. He lived during the first century A.D., and was a compiler of information rather than a practicing physician. His work on medicine is the only surviving section of a comprehensive encyclopedia of knowledge that he produced, or at least planned. His work on medicine is systematic, thorough and highly informative, and also is written in classic literary Latin. The medical practices that he describes and the doctrines that he advances are improvements in several ways beyond the Hippocratic level and many of his concepts and explications are basic to modern medicine.

Surgical instruments, unfortunately, have not survived well over long periods of time and, therefore, archaeological excavations of earlier sites have not revealed many. The more complete and impressive arrays come from later sites within the Christian era. Three are noteworthy for the range and preservation of the items which they contained. Pompeii and Herculaneum, which preserved many artifacts through the sealing effect of the volcanic ash from Mt. Vesuvius, have yielded a number of well preserved surgical instruments, symbolizing the state of the art as of A.D. 62. Some of these demonstrate the mechanical ingenuity and the skillful execution of Roman craftsmen in producing devices well improved beyond the Hippocratic stage of design. The Romans added their metal working and mechanical capabilities to the design of earlier items and produced many instruments of such quality that they were ancestral to those of Renaissance and modern production.

One noteworthy cache of surgical instruments was in the discovery of an ancient Roman military hospital site at Baden in Germany, excavated in 1893. Many instruments were found, including 120 probes as well as cauteries and cases for instruments. Another find was of a grave in Paris of the second or early third century A.D., that of a physician who was buried with a bronze pot containing much of his professional equipment. (This calls forth speculation as to the possible emotional involvements of the doctor with the implements of his profession as interpreted by his surviving relatives who perhaps ordered the inhumation of all items related to the sensitive manipulations of his operating fingers.) This bronze vessel contained forceps, bleeding cups, probes and knife blades, all typical of the current Roman practice at the time.

There are many occasional finds that have brought to light Roman technology of the early post-Christian period. The total impression that we can derive from a study of such collections is that Western surgery is a continuum, with numerous breaks and periods of retrogression, but with an overall progress from primitive Greco-Roman battlefield surgery and domestic medication toward the achievements of twentieth century medicine and surgery.

With reference to what can be justifiably conjectured, the scope of the pre-Hippocratic physician's surgical practice was probably something like this. Traumatic surgery was probably his major specialty, not only from military injuries but from sports casualties resulting from the violent and exhausting games and diversions of the Greeks (Phillips 1973: 96). The physician would have had to deal with sprains, dislocations and fractures as well as with weapon wounds. In these areas he was no doubt reasonably competent as a result of his extensive experience. It is questionable whether he would have been able to trephine the skull in a clean cut and efficient manner. He certainly was able to elevate bone fragments and cleanse and bandage the wound. He probably opened abscesses and tumors, and perhaps burned out tumors by cauterization.

Some of the doctor's practice was perhaps in the care of hunting misadventures such as snakebites, claw wounds, contusions and other results of the pursuit of game animals over a precipitous terrain. The ligation of blood vessels to arrest hemorrhaging is first mentioned by Celsus in the first century A.D. (Ackerknecht 1971: 96). Amputation would have been unknown, since it was not practiced by the Hippocratic surgeons. There is mention, however, of a natural "blackening" where a dead limb, because of poor circulation can become mummified and fall off, a natural amputation that was given some surgical attention (Majno 1975: 191-192).

The pre-Hippocratic surgeon probably had considerable practice in dealing with female disorders. He would have made vaginal examinations and performed curettage (Milne 1907: 157). Normal childbirth was managed by midwives, but in the case of difficulties the doctor would have been consulted. He may have manually effected version of the fetus in some cases. Obstetrical forceps would not come into use until the seventeenth century A.D. Since there is no mention of Caesarian section in the Hippocratic corpus, it was probably unknown during earlier times in Greece, although it was performed on slaves as early as the second millenium B.C. in Mesopotamia (Biggs 1969: 100-101). It is apparently referred to in the *Corpus Juris* of Justinian of the sixth century B.C., which forbids the interment of a pregnant woman before the offspring has been cut from her (Oppenheim 1960: 293). On occasion the surgeon probably performed embryoctony.

The Hippocratic documents mention surgical efforts to treat congenital club foot in children. Bending the foot bones "inwards" and bandaging are indicated, with a sole of leather or lead attached outside the bandage (Phillips 1973: 102). This fairly simple orthopedic manipulation could well have been known in pre-Hippocratic times.

There is some mystery as to how far back in medical history the operation of lithotomy for the removal of urinary calculi was performed. It has been stated that Egyptians were skilled in the operation (Baas 1971: 18) and it was apparently well known to the early doctors of India. Meges of Sidon, who lived during the first century B.C., is credited with inventing instruments for cutting stones (Berdoe 1893: 215). Hippocrates alludes to lithotomy in a negative way in his famous physician's oath. The physician avers that he will not perform the operation but will leave it to "men who are practitioners of this work." There is some doubt as to the meaning of this passage. It may imply that lithotomy operations were, along with castration, considered the work of empirics rather than respectable surgeons (Castiglioni 1975: 145, 154). The somewhat mild flavor of the phrase "practitioners of this work," who may have been regarded as quacks, is perhaps to be explained by the lack of any clear legal demarcation between legitimate and charlatanic medicine in ancient Greece (Jones 1946: 34).

There is some doubt that lithotomy operations were performed by pre-Hippocratic Greek surgeons of good reputation. The need for the operation was unquestionably great among the populace, but the fact that it was apparently considered unworthy of a legitimate surgeon would perhaps indicate that while it was occasionally performed by poorly trained individuals it was not perfected and was often unsuccessful. The Roman physicians apparently were well versed in the technique of the operation since Celsus describes perineal lithotomy in considerable detail and with good understanding (Wangensteen and Wangensteen 1979: 212). Yet the highly competent and greatly respected surgeon of his time, the fourteenth century French physician Guy de Chauliac, would not perform lithotomy operations, although he operated for cataract and rupture (Garrison 1929: 157; Singer and Underwood 1962: 83).

In general dental surgery was largely undeveloped by the Greeks and Romans. An exception, however, was in the prosthetic dentistry of the Etruscans, who preceded the Romans in many parts of Italy prior to the fifth century B.C. They were expert in gold working and inserted artificial teeth held in position by bands of gold (Major 1954: 155-157). Missing teeth were replaced by the patient's own extracted teeth, animal teeth, the teeth of slaves or teeth carved of bone or ivory. Bridges of gold were made to fit around the crowns of rooted teeth. The teeth of dead persons were not used since this was probably contrary to the religious laws of the time or would have been repulsive to the wearer. In one specimen found in the necropolis at Tarquinii an ox tooth was inserted in a gold appliance anchored to adjoining teeth. This took the place of two central incisors. The ox tooth replacement was grooved to make it resemble the two missing teeth (Guerini 1969: 71-73).

Among the Romans the only form of dental surgery practiced seems to have been tooth extraction. Celsus mentions that when extracting a tooth with a large cavity, the hole should be filled with lint or lead in order to prevent the tooth from being crushed by the forceps (Guerini 1969: 87). There was apparently no class of dental surgeons, and there is no Latin word for dentist.*

Surgery in Ancient India

While outside the corridor of evolution of Western medicine, the early development of surgical technology in India is impressive, although it apparently had little influence on later developments in scientific medicine.

In India surgery and other aspects of medical knowledge were strangely inconsistent. Much early Hindu medicine involved witchcraft and demonology, and anatomical knowledge and physiological theory were fanciful and inaccurate. The human body was thought to have three hundred bones and five hundred muscles, while air was said to be the basic physiological principle. Diseases were classified as natural and supernatural in source, and over one thousand were identified. Susruta defined 66 diseases of the oral cavity and 5 of the earlobe. In contrast to this welter of folkloristic imagination, a high level of skill in surgery and in the design of surgical instruments was achieved. Eight techniques were cited in Indian operative surgery: incision, excision, scraping, puncturing, probing, extraction, provoking secretion and suturing (Ackerknecht 1968: 42).

Classical Indian medicine developed between 700 B.C. and 200 B.C. reaching its peak around 200 B.C. The refinement and elaboration of Hindu surgical methods is set forth in the Susruta (the name of both the work and the author), a Brahmanical text of the fifth century A.D. In this it is indicated that there were 121 different surgical instruments in use including not only knives, probes, shears, forceps and needles, but also trocars, catheters and bougies. The instruments were well made and those with blades were kept sharp and polished (Thompson 1942: 17). Steel was probably introduced quite early in India (Forbes 1954: 597). The range of operations was impressive, since it included amputations, cauterization, lithotomy, cataract operations, Caesarian section, and, when needed to save the mother, embryoctony (Baas 1971: 46).

---

*Nor is there a classical Greek word for dentist. The modern Greek term ὀδοντίατρος is merely a late convenient coinage meaning "doctor of teeth."

Their methods of teaching surgical techniques were ingenious and efficient. They taught the ways of handling tissue through exercises on plants, on models consisting of animal bladders and sacks filled with water or mud, also on dead animals. Bandaging was taught on life sized dolls stuffed with linen.

The operation of rhinoplasty, the rebuilding of the nose through plastic surgery, was well developed. Amputation of the nose was a common punishment for adultery, and there were numerous patients who sought to have their appearance restored. Another well perfected operation was the plastic repair of split earlobes that had been ripped in two through wearing heavy earrings (Majno 1975: 288-292).

With the spread of Buddhism a doctrinal preoccupation with the sanctity of animals made animal dissection and animal experimentation impossible, and along with this there was a growing abhorrence of blood and disease. These forces brought the development of surgery to a halt and furthered the retrogression of the art. Surgical skills early reached a high level in India, but anatomic knowledge and physiological understanding never advanced much beyond a primitive folkloristic stage. Surgical practice deteriorated to a few operations performed by village healers with little background and limited training.

There is an important contrast between Greek and Hindu medicine and surgery. Although the Hindus achieved a striking advancement in the techniques of surgery, their theory of medicine was heavily involved with magic and supernaturalism. The Greeks, while not as adept as the Hindus in their operative techniques, achieved the separation of medicine from religion that was never accomplished by the Hindus. This religious association kept Hindu healing procedures from advancing toward a science.

In dealing with early surgery one factor must be emphasized. The surgeon's success in treating his patients was largely tilted in his favor by the fact that most of his patients were young. The average life expectancy at birth in early Greece was around twenty years (Coon and Hunt 1963: 45). In addition the clean air, the lack of urban congestion and the fact that healing procedures were largely individual rather than in hospitalized communities all could have contributed to his success.

CHAPTER 3

ABORIGINAL AFRICA AND ASIA

WHILE SOME of the peoples of Western Europe were emerging from a prescientific toward a scientific level of medical knowledge and techniques, there were many who, in parts of Europe, Africa, Asia, Oceania and the New World, were developing prescientific healing traditions and surgical methods that have continued into recent and contemporary times. The procedures employed in these cases have often been brutal, clumsy and ineffective, but some have been efficient and have improved the lot of suffering patients.

At this point we are detached from the main current of the evolution of medicine in the trend initiated by the Greeks through using rigorous logic, experimentation and recorded observation to describe and alleviate human disorders. The peoples considered from now on will be aboriginals of lesser developed cultures, mostly pre-literate, some of whom developed a degree of healing knowledge and skill through empirical observation that was passed down by memory in families and professional coteries. Such methods at times have been helpful to the patient, but many have been disastrous. Some of the empirical healing methods were of psychosomatic value and some have involved useful herbs and other medicaments that have been incorporated into present day pharmacopoeias. Many of the surgical methods, if they can be broadly called that, have been nothing more than decorative or symbolic body mutilation, demon expelling devices or punishment for the transgression of tribal mores. The surgical methods of aboriginal peoples had one thing in

50

common: they were usually administered with dramatic authority and supernatural aegis and accordingly had powerful suggestive impact.

Several reasons for backwardness in medical and surgical achievement among many native peoples could be cited. Primarily such peoples had no tradition in their culture that stressed the value of the systematic gathering and classification of knowledge in any area. Also many, but not all of such peoples have been preliterate, which prevented the recording of observed data and placed the entire burden of transmitting knowledge on the memory of individuals which could have been imperfect and could have deteriorated with time.

A third and highly important reason was that in most of these cultures supernatural concepts were a vital part of the thought processes of the people; and body disasters were attributed to the anger of spirits or the presence of evil demons in the body and were treated through expiation and exorcism. This framework of explanation left no room for naturalistic healing procedures. A lack of manual skill and dexterity can rarely be cited since many aboriginal peoples, outstandingly in Africa, have displayed great technical ability in ceramics, weaving and metal working.

In aboriginal Africa, except for a few areas, surgery was little developed beyond minor manipulations or ritual and cosmetic mutilations. In contrast herbal medicine was at times complex and quite often effective. The Zulus, with little surgical knowledge or skill, knew as many as 700 plants with medicinal applications and the average native doctor was apparently able to identify and make use of over 200 plants (Bryant 1970: 84). In contrast to the usual undeveloped state of native African surgery, the Masai surgeon of East Africa was able to perform a number of difficult surgical operations including amputations and the suturing of blood vessels. Circumcision, which, when properly performed, requires considerable surgical expertise, was done widely and successfully in Africa, often by peoples who did not show a comparable degree of proficiency in operations for a healing purpose. A considerable amount of crude and inhumane body mutilation was done for judicial and punitive reasons.

Selecting from which viewpoint to discuss African aboriginal surgery creates a problem. Many of the practices, particularly in north and east Africa, were strongly influenced by Arabian and Greek through Arabian traditions. The strictly aboriginal concepts and practices have been a combination of empirical knowledge, based on many generations of experience passed down in familial lines combined with folklore and shamanistic performance, and in some cases include a considerable degree of manual skill. A certain amount of tissue cutting, drug therapy and psychotherapy were all involved, often undoubtedly with a beneficial effect on an ailing patient. The strictly surgical aspect of this complex cannot be extracted reasonably from the other elements; yet since our central theme is surgery our main discussion will be the operative surgical methods used although it must be borne in mind that herbs, ritual and suggestion may be highly important elements in native healing procedure.

Bloodletting

Bloodletting is an almost universal minor surgical expedient utilized by peoples of both primitve and advanced culture status. The conditions thought to have been relieved by the practice are numerous. Headaches, pneumonia, pleurisy, fevers and practically all human disorders from time to time have been treated by this means. Galen claimed that he had saved himself and others from the plague in Asia by venesection (Thorndike 1923, vol. 1: 125). There have been a number of proposed theoretical reasons for its use. It has been thought that an excess of blood causes disease, and also that spirits that cause disease can be placated by offerings of blood. Under most circumstances it can be assumed with good reason that bleeding was a deterrent to the recovery of an ailing patient, although perhaps at times bloodletting could have been a useful decongestant and possibly could have provided relief. Such occasional instances of value in the procedure, through overemphasis and lack of critical evaluation, could have led to the widespread practice of phlebotomy.

The idea of bloodletting became a part of many cultures and has survived well into the modern period of medical history. It reached its peak of popularity during the nineteenth century when, in 1883, it is said that 41 million leeches were imported into France for the purpose of bloodletting and that patients in hospitals were bled before they were examined by physicians (Singer and Underwood 1962: 282).

Bloodletting is a common feature of primitive surgery in Africa where it is done to relieve many types of aches, pains, and regional disorders. It has also been thought to give strength and precision to body action in hunting and warlike activities. Among the native peoples of Morocco the vein of the left arm is opened to relieve congestion of the spleen and one in the right arm for congestion in the liver. A statement of the doctrine involved in Moroccan bloodletting has been given as follows:

> The body is divided into five parts that are tributary for bloodletting to the frontal vein, to the radials and to the veins of the ankle. The vein is opened in that part of the body where the bloodletting is most useful. In performing major bloodletting it is necessary to open the five veins (Dubie quoted by Lillico 1940: 138).

There were several methods of letting blood from the body in primitive practice:

(1) **Scarification:** This is merely the slashing of the skin that produces a flow of blood.

(2) **Cupping:** This is quite common in Africa and apparently replaced an earlier technique of using scarification alone. It is essentially a method of accelerating the blood flow produced by scarification.

(3) **Venesection:** This invovles opening a specific blood vessel, commonly a vein. It occurs in the Americas, but occasionally in Africa.

(4) **Leeching:** Leeches are attached to the patient to draw blood, an ingenious effort to engage the services of another organism to combat human illness. It earliest occurrence was apparently in Asia.

The terminology in this area is somewhat confused. The general term of *bloodletting* refers to any artificial effort to release blood from the body. It includes crude slashing or scarification as well as more refined methods. *Phlebotomy*, from the derivation of the word, could apply to the opening of either a vein or an artery, but current usage limits its use mainly to the sectioning of a vein. *Venesection* or *venetomy* refers specifically to the opening of a vein. *Arteriotomy* applies to the opening of an artery.

Native African procedures in general have not been aimed at specific blood vessels but were merely the cutting through of the skin and slashing any vessels that lay in the path of the knife. Bloodletting by scarification alone is a slow method of extracting blood from the body and is often accelerated by cupping. The essential procedure in cupping is to place a cup, made usually from a horn but sometimes made of clay or metal, over the scarified part. The horn is cut so that there is an opening at the tip and it is sucked upon by the operator which reduces the atmospheric pressure in the cup and this increases the blood flow. The small opening is often sealed with wax or some other substance making the horn adhere through suction to the patient's body. It is usually left there until the horn is filled with a quantity of blood that the operator considers adequate.

The cupping practice of the Lango of Uganda, central Africa, is explained as follows:

> The following procedure is observed in bleeding. The cupping horn has a hole at the tip and is applied to the affected part, whereupon the operator sucks until the blood collects under the skin, when the horn is removed and several small incisions are made on the skin. The horn is then returned to position (the hole in the tip having first been covered with a leaf of a plant, *inege*, to prevent the blood reaching the mouth), and the operator sucks the blood into the horn. This operation does not necessitate the services of a professional *ajoka*, or witch-doctor, but a fee of one chicken is payable to any operator engaged outside of the family of the invalid; an *ajoka* is necessary, however, to remove pus from boils by sucking direct without a horn. (Driberg 1923: 56).

In Africa cupping is quite general and has probably replaced an earlier practice of scarification (Ackerknecht 1947: 29). Cupping, while extensively done by the Greeks and Romans, seems to have been uncommon among most aboriginal peoples other than the Africans and some American Indians. Cupping is recorded among the peoples of Africa from the Berbers of the north to the Hottentots and Bantu peoples of the south.

Scarification followed by cupping is a common remedy for pain, particularly headache, chest pains and back pain. The procedure of incision is often quite specific. Among the Wayao of southwest Africa six small incisions are made with a triangular knife. The same knife is used in tattooing and circumcision (Stannus 1922: 289). With the Ba-Yaka of the lower Congo the cupping horn is left in place for around one half hour (Torday and Joyce 1906: 50). Among the Zulus for paralysis an incision is made on the patient's shadow on the ground and continued up the unaffected side of his body. The following day the process is repeated on the other side of his body. The bark of the *Xanthoxylon capense* tree is rubbed into the incisions (Bryant 1970: 69). At times dry cupping is used. In this the skin is not broken and the blood is engorged through suction in the region where the cup is applied.

Wet cupping, cupping after slashing, is sometimes an accompaniment of shamanistic healing. The South African healer will sometimes draw blood from his patient by slashing and cupping and then carefully examine the extracted blood. He may remove an ant, beetle or other insect from the blood and then confidently announce that the cause of the patient's illness has been removed and that he will recover (McDonald 1890: 274).

While scarification is often done for bloodletting it is also carried out for other purposes. It may be done for decoration and for symbolic reasons. Lines, cruciform designs and other elements may be created. Among the Lango of Uganda the pattern radiates from the breastbone over the shoulder and upper arms. The designs apparently have no symbolic significance and are purely decorative. The Lango method of creating the scars is as follows: A bent needle or a sharp thorn is used to raise a fold of skin which is then cut off with a sharp knife. Sesame oil mixed with red chalk is rubbed into the wound. A ceremonial form of scarification follows a hostile encounter during which a victim is killed. The victorious attacker then scarifies himself with a number of slashes. It has been suggested that this ceremonial slashing of the body is a form of offering to the spirit of the person killed to keep it from seeking vengeance on the killer. It has also been proposed that the decorative form of scarification may be a secularized deterioration of the cerermonial form (Driberg 1923: 51-52).

Among some African peoples a form of skin cutting is used as tribal markings on boys. With the Lilawa of Nigeria characteristic parallel linear cuts are made on the face and in the case of a first born child on the upper arms and forearms. This is done by a barber with a special knife when the child is three months old. Girls at between seven and ten years of age are subjected to cicitrization on various parts of the body. It is said to be done to remove bad blood and to further the beauty of the girl (Harris 1938: 132-133).

The use of incisions in the opening of abscesses and tumors is varied. A number of peoples do this by means of thorns and knives but others leave such conditions to a natural culmination. Sometimes the attitude toward such tissue manipulation was quite inconsistent. The Wayao of East Africa leave all tumors and abscesses untouched, but cut off accessory digits in infancy. The same people have a belief that fevers in newborn children are caused by hymenal caruncles on the mother and these are cut off by old medicine women and the blood allowed to drip on the mother (Stannus 1922: 287).

Incision in the neck and removal of swollen lymph nodes are reported by a number of observers (Ackerknecht 1947: 31). This is done to relieve a condition brought on by the African sleeping sickness disease, *African trypanosomiasis*, which is characterized by fever, regional swelling and morbid enlargement of the lymph nodes.

In treating fever the Thonga of South Africa make incisions in the temporal region with a razor and apply a cupping horn over the incisions.

Sex Organ Mutilation

Excision of parts of the external sex organs is a widespread form of minor surgery in Africa and in many other parts of the world. *Circumcision* involves the cutting away of the male prepuce after it has been drawn forward over the glans penis. This is done in varying degrees of severity as examples will indicate.

Circumcision has been widespread in native Africa. However, a number of tribal groups that formerly followed the practice have dropped it. The Zulus and most of the peoples of Bechuanaland have abandoned it. On the other hand it has gained ground among the Venda and is practiced by a great number of South and East African peoples (Schapera 1953: 100). Tribes not greatly separated in distance have had quite different cultural characteristics, including adherence to the practice of circumcision. The Bayaka of the lower Congo practice circumcision while the Bambala of the not greatly distant Rhodesian area do not. The Bayaka practice scarification, while it is rare among the Bambala, and cannibalism is abhorred by the Bayaka but often practiced by the Bambala (Torday and Joyce 1906: 40).

Circumcision reached Africa through the Islamic world, although circumcision is not mentioned in the Koran (Turner 1915: 134). All Bantu races were formerly circumcised, but a Zulu king Jobe ordered the practice stopped because the complex rituals involved interfered with his military encampments (Turner 1915: 134). Now practically all of the Zulu races are uncircumcised.

The operation is often performed with considerable care and skill. The following description of circumcision among the Bambuti Pygmies of the central Congo suggests the gravity which surrounds the rite and the skill in performing the operation by a people whose surgical accomplishments in other respects are minimal.

> The first three boys were then brought in quick succession to the initiation camp and circumcised. Each was carried in on the back of the village headman (a MuBira) and placed on the trestle. The boy put one arm around the headman, and one around his father. Other men, negroes and pygmies, crowded around to assist in holding him still. The two operators knelt in front, holding the boys' legs open, and Andre operated with a series of eight or nine steady, deliberate cuts, inspecting the wound carefully after each cut. The actual operation took four minutes in each case. During the operation the boys all maintained silence for the first cut or two, but after that they were smothered by the hands and arms of the onlookers to prevent them from crying. The first boy was given a whistle to blow during the operation, and he was frequently rapped on the head by the onlookers, using their fists or their knuckles.
>
> Immediately after the last cut the wound was washed and wrapped in a leaf containing a medicine prepared from powdered roots and banana-skins. Black paste was smeared on the forehead and nose, and each boy was carried to a log on which he was made to sit, legs apart, while the blood dripped into a leaf cup placed on the ground. No sooner had the first boy sat down than

he was made to learn his first initiation song (Turnbull 1957: 194).

A more painful operation is performed by the Kipsiki or Lumbwa tribe of Kenya. Here the foreskin is pulled forward and cut off. The glans penis is pulled forward. The outer skin of the penis is pressed back and the tissue beneath this outer skin is pared away. The outer skin is then brought forward and fastened by two thorns, piercing the outer skin from right to left. The operation is accompanied by severe pain and suppuration and in time the thorn needles rot away (Barton 1923: 54).

Among the Berbers of Algeria the rite is also a solemn affair and the procedures are more complicated. Again the operator is not a surgeon but a ritual functionary. Care is taken to keep demons away during the operation. An attendant holds salt in his hand and makes seven rotatory movements around the patient's body. Guns are fired at the moment of cutting. A knobbed stick is forced against the glans penis of the patient, the foreskin being drawn over the knob. This is secured by a piece of string, firmly tied. The foreskin is removed by a quick downward cut with an ordinary knife. After the operation a raw egg is opened at one end and pressed upon the patient's penis, perhaps a symbol of fertility. Juniper leaves and melted butter are applied to the wound (Hilton-Simpson 1922: 60-61).

The instruments used in circumcision and other operations on the genital organs vary with the available resources and ingenuity of the operators. Chipped stone was perhaps the earliest form, having been used by prehistoric man, and being employed in more recent times occasionally as a symbolic survival. Most of the African peoples who were early in developing the technology of iron working, made knives and razors that were suitable. Other peoples have used broken glass, mussel shells and splinters of bamboo. The people of Tonga dispense with instruments, tearing the foreskin with the fingers of the operator (Hastings 1913: III 650).

Surgery on the external sex organs in primitive cultures is usually not done by surgeons, and the operators are often regarded as minor religious officials and are subject to taboos (Crosse-Upcott 1959: 181). Operations on females are often done by older women. The operators who perform these operations are rarely concerned with healing activities.

The reasons for circumcision and other sex organ excisions are lost in antiquity and are obscured by cultural diffusion. A number of theories of origin have been proposed, some of which may have applied in certain areas but not in others. The most commonly cited explanations have been as follows:

Hygiene: This is the justification for the modern surgical practice of circumcision, but is unlikely for peoples of prescientific culture status since most of these have vague and limited concepts of infection and the need for cleanliness.

Preparation for sexual life and the enhancement of sexual satisfaction and efficiency: This has dubious physiological justification.

Sacrificial offerings: this involves offering a part of the body to save the whole through the gratification of spirits. This is possibly applicable among some American Indian and a few African peoples, notably the West African Yoruba and Ewe.

Tests of endurance: This is somewhat doubtful since ability to withstand pain is a feature of many aboriginal rites, and circumcision would not appear to be more important in this regard than many more exacting ordeals.

Magic of a released constriction: The theory is that the foreskin is a presumed constriction that mythically obstructs growth and development and therefore to remove it is an aid to successful procreation (Flack 1939: 28). This is a magical hypothesis and can be evaluated only in relation to the other supernatural concepts of the culture involved.

A political indicator of tribal unity and class distinction: This has had varying applications and may well have been the most prevalent explanation. It clearly applied among the ancient Hebrews along with the concept of a covenant with Yahweh (Genesis 17: 9-11).

Numerous other explanations have been offered but the above listed hypotheses incorporate most of the others (Hastings 1913: 664-666).

A more radical phase of the mutilation of the male external sex organs is castration, *orchiectomy* or *orchidectomy*, the removal of the testes. A few peoples, including those of the Loyalty Islands, the Carolines, Tonga and also the Hottentots, have followed the strange practice of excising one testicle (Ackerknecht 1947: 35). This operation, *monorchiectomy*, has been practiced on practically all the males of the Hottentots and Caroline Islanders (McKenzie 1927: 373), but seems to have had little effect on the fecundity of the population. More drastic than castration has been the excision of the penis, *penectomy* or *phallectomy*. This has occurred mainly in the Orient.

An operation applied to both males and females is infibulation. The purpose of the operation is to prevent coitus. For the male this is usually the insertion of a ring or pin at the end of the penis or the partial stitching closed of the opening at the end. For females it involves the stitching together of the labia majora, and is done early in adolescent life to prevent coitus until marriage, at which time the stitches are removed. This may be done several times in the life of a woman in order to prevent sexual intercourse during the absence of her husband. This practice occurs mainly in Ethiopia and Somaliland and is an example of the rare use of ligatures in native African surgery (McKenzie 1927: 376).

Not all circumcision has been deeply involved with ritual. Female circumcision is in general less connected with religious doctrine than that on males. Some people, such as the Afikpo Ibo of Eastern Nigeria circumcise their boys with little ritual in early infancy but initiate them in their late teens with rites that involve elaborate tests of strength and courage (Ottenburg 1965: 23). The Gula and Lendu and their relatives practice circumcision, but the Sara, some Mamvu and Madi use no genital mutilation and extract central incisor teeth as an initiatory rite. The Lango of Uganda do not circumcise their boys although there is considerable phymosis among them, a condition that involves the narrowing of the opening of the prepuce that prevents it from being drawn back over the glans, an unfavorable condition that can be relieved by circumcision.

Hemostasis and Counterirritation

Attempts to arrest the flow of blood from a wound or surgical incision have been varied and usually inefficient in aboriginal African surgical practice. Tourniquets were known and used by some peoples, but others, even those who understand wet cupping after incisions, were ignorant of their use (Stannus 1922: 289). Cauterization was known and used to stop blood flow by some African peoples and was also used in other ways. Neck tumors were cauterized in Rhodesia and cauterization was used as a cure for pleurisy and pneumonia in Uganda. Cauterization was often applied in an area of pain. Cauterization perhaps had a folkloristic origin for its supposed efficacy. The worship of fire was quite general among earlier peoples and the application of the cauterizing iron that had been withdrawn from a fire perhaps was thought to bring this mysterious power to aid in curing the patient's ailment. Cauterization was certainly given more significance than its role as a hemostatic agent would have justified and it seems to have been at times used as a counterirritant.

Among the Dinkas counterirritation is the basis of most treatments. Headache is treated by tying a cord around the head, and bronchitis and chest pains are dealt with by tying a cord around the thorax. The flesh is cut with knives over the seat of a pain and cupping is applied over the scarified surface. Also cauterization or "firing" with hot irons is used (Cummins 1904: 156).

The Thonga of South Africa use a novel method of cauterization for pleurisy. The operator heats an iron hoe red hot. He then smears medicine on the sole of his foot and places it on the hot hoe blade. He then places his heated foot on the patient's body which is blistered where the foot has been applied. The callused foot of the operator is not injured (Harley 1941: 227).

In treating ragged wounds the Banyankole of East Central Africa heat a spear point and work it inside the wound to stop the bleeding and burn out any unhealthy tissue.

Dislocations and Fractures

Dislocations are often reduced quite effectively by aboriginal Africans. The Hottentots rub the joint area with fat and vigorously move the limb up and down. Some of the South African peoples dig a hole in the ground in which the arm or leg of the patient is buried and firmly held by the compaction of the earth. The body of the patient is then pulled until the bones forming the joint are restored to their proper relationship (Kidd 1904: 136).

A number of African peoples are fairly successful in dealing with fractures. The Zulus, before any contact with Europeans, made splints of split dog's bones bound on each side of a fractured limb. They also made incisions in the skin in the area of the fracture and rubbed in a powder made from the dried root of certain herbs that were thought to have healing power (Bryant 1970: 77-78). The Tanala of Madagascar use heavy bandages but no splints.

Amputations

Amputation for medical purposes is rare among native Africans. It is sometimes done as a ritual symbol, particularly of mourning. Hottentots occasionally amputate a finger by first tying the finger with sinew above the joint and then cut through the flesh and ligaments with a knife. A Hottentot widow who marries a second time must have the distal joint of her little finger amputated. Another joint is removed each time she marries (Gould and Pyle 1956: 746). The Masai of the Lake Victoria Nyanza region, who are noteworthy for their efficient level of aboriginal surgery, tie a limb firmly above the area of the amputation and cut the member off with a single blow of a sharp sword (Harley 1941: 222).

A possible case of amputation of a lower limb at the thigh is reported for the Yaka of West Africa where the patient was suffering from destruction of tissue caused by the sand flea (Bartels 1893: 293). Such major amputations are quite rare, but occasional amputations of a finger or a supernumerary digit in infancy are more frequent.

An incident is reported in Swaziland, South Africa where a man suffering from a painful corn on his toe amputated a joint of his own toe with a chisel in order to end his suffering from the corn (Kidd 1904: 288). In general amputation is not attempted in the areas under the Islamic influence, since Moslem doctrine forbids it.

Major Operations

Abdominal operations were rarely performed in aboriginal Africa. While there are reports of a surgeon removing surgically a fetus after a mother has died, true Caesarian section is rare. The only area where there seems to have been competency in this operation has been Uganda in East Central Africa. An unusual and classical case was reported by a scientifically trained British observer who had seen the operation in progress in 1879. The essentials of the operative technique were as follows:

The patient had been semi-intoxicated with banana wine. She was placed upon an inclined bed and held down by bands of bark cloth around her thorax and held at her ankles by an assistant. The operating surgeon made a rapid cut on the midline of the abdomen from a little above the pubes to just below the umbilicus. The assistant held the abdominal walls apart with two fingers of both hands. The child was given to another assistant and the cord was cut. Some use of cauterization was made to reduce hemorrhage. The placenta was removed and the surgeon kept a firm pressue on the uterus until it was contracted. The uterine wall was not sutured but a grass mat was secured over the wound. Finally seven thin iron pins were inserted in the flesh on either side of the incision and drawn together with a string made from bark cloth. A paste was applied, then a warmed banana leaf and a cloth bandage. The wound was dressed and from the third morning on the pins were progressively removed and after eleven days the wound was healed and the mother and child appeared to be in a healthy state (Felkin 1884: 928-929).

Trephination

Probably the most exacting surgical operation attempted by native African doctors has been trephining the skull, and this has been limited to a few tribal groups only. The Berbers and Kabyles of northern Africa developed skill in the trephining operation and it apparently was known among the now extinct Guanches of the Canary Islands off the northwest coast of Africa (Hooton 1925: 154). The Kisii in Kenya, East Africa, and the Tende somewhat further south and into Tanganyika have been carefully observed and photographed in regard to their trephining practice.* Numerous other

---

*A motion picture of the Kisii operation in progress, sponsored by a West German chemical manufacturing house, was released in 1964 with the title "Maganga." It was critically reviewed on several grounds (Dauer and Karolyi 1970: 138-144), but defended for its scientific value in a further review (Schadewalt 1970: 289-298). The latter reiew includes an interesting summary of comments and literature on native trephining in Africa.

peoples are rumored to have trephined skulls of the living, and occasional trephined skulls have been reported although there is some
uncertainty in distinguishing between trephination and cauterization of the skull, the latter having been widely practiced (Margetts
1967: 680-682). The Kisii procedure is described as follows:

> The scalp is incised in a linear or cruciate manner over the site
> of the headache and the flaps if need be are retracted by the
> fingers of assistants. As a rule nothing is added to the wound, but
> occasionally, a medicine (unidentified) is sprinkled in the site to
> assuage pain, and sometimes an agent like charcoal or local pres-
> sure is applied for haemostasis. Any fragments of bone, foreign
> bodies or clotted blood are removed, and any discolored bone or
> fracture line is removed by scraping the skull with a sharp scrap-
> ing knife having an acutely curved tip, curved to avoid punc-
> turing the dura and brain. The scraping is usually continued
> until the inner table is pierced and the brain membranes ex-
> posed. Less frequently a saw is employed to make the hole. Most
> operators are able to distinguish the cranial sutures from fracture
> lines, and seem to realize the danger of puncturing the dura,
> though in ignorance this is sometimes done in the case of sub-
> dural haematoma. Usually, both inner and outer tables of the
> skull are holed, but not always. After sufficient bone has been re-
> moved, the wound is washed with water. One *omobari* is said to
> have spewed water from his mouth onto the wound—no doubt an
> effective stream but not very aseptic.
>
> Fat or butter may then be applied with a feather or other ap-
> plicator. Sometimes herbal medicines are added to promote heal-
> ing. The wound is usually allowed to heal by granulation; the
> scalp may rarely be sutured, in the common native-fashion with
> figure-of-eight sutures over thorns. The operation is said to cause
> only very little pain, except initially as the soft tissues are cut and
> retracted. Anaesthesia is not employed (Margetts 1967: 683-
> 684).

The operation usually takes from one to four hours and is accompanied by a certain amount of preliminary supernatural ministra-
tion. The instruments used, of which there are a number, are made
of iron, rather well fashioned, but fitted with crude wooden handles.
The success of the operation is notable, mortality being estimated at
no more than five percent. In the Kisii area the operation is per-

formed mainly to relieve headaches following a head injury that may or may not have involved skull fracture.

The development of a competent trephining operation in northern Africa among the Berbers, Kabylea and possibly also the Guanches, can probably be explained by the closeness of these peoples to the Arabs and Europeans through whom Greek medical principles and practices could in some measure have been transmitted. It is much more difficult to explain the occurrence of trephining among the Kisii, Tende and Masai whose much greater distance from Europe would have made the diffusion of such a specific cultural achievement less likely. It would perhaps appear that a combination of ingenuity, skill and the previous development of iron technology all could have been contributing factors.

In a review of the surgical concepts and procedures of native Africa it is interesting to note in particular certain cultures that are the most north in location and are accordingly the most likely to reflect the influence of European and Arabian concepts. The remote peoples of Algeria give us a valuable indication of the status of surgical knowledge and skills in the region that lies close to Europe and was influenced by Moslem culture but reflects certain ancient aboriginal practices.

The native surgeon of ancient Berber stock, according to his own evaluation of his craft, has achieved remarkable results, superior to those of Western doctors. An example is in the avoidance of amputation that is dreaded most vehemently by the Moslems for supposed dire implications in the next world. The terrified patient, who has been advised by a European doctor that amputation of an arm or leg is inevitable, has often appealed to a native doctor who has relieved his condition without amputation (Hilton-Simpson 1922: 12-13). That the patient recovers without amputation can perhaps be explained by the innate vigor of the patient and the powerful psychotherapeutic impact of the native doctor's methods, notwithstanding his crude and unsterile technique.

The Berber surgeon is proud of his deft skill and his delicate manipulation of his patient. Notwithstanding the lack of cleanliness and disregard of contamination that is revolting to a person accustomed to the techniques of Western medicine, the native doctor has often attempted difficult surgical tasks and attained remarkable results.

He usually operates without anaesthesia.

The outstanding major operation of the native doctor is trephining the skull (Hilton-Simpson 1922: 30 et seq.). This operation is performed solely to relieve the effects of blows on the head and has no supernatural and animistic implications. In cases where the injury is small, scraping is all that is done, but in larger traumatized areas there is usually a combination of drilling and sawing. The drill is a specially made instrument with a wooden handle and usually with a flat iron blade brought to a shouldered point. The shouldering is for the purpose of keeping the point from entering the bone of the skull too deeply, since the surgeon is always very careful not to penetrate the dura mater. Other types of point are used, some with three points, the middle one acting as a guide and the outer two cutting the circular groove. The drill is manipulated by rotating the shaft between the palms of the hands and used to bore either a single hole as a starting point for the saw, or to produce a series of holes that are later joined by saw cuts, after which the bone segment is elevated and removed. The operation usually requires around one and one half hours. The circular trephine is not used. The scalp is not stitched and usually no attempt is made to replace the removed bone or insert any covering plate or replacement. The operation is frequently performed, and apparently with a high degree of success. Islamic surgeons in North Africa are careful not to damage the brain and its coverings and to avoid cutting through sutures since these are believed to be the patient's destiny written by the hand of Allah (Rogers, L. 1930: 498).

Native surgeons are competent in setting fractures and have several types of splints, some being made of wooden slats cut in a curved form to fit the member. Some splints are made of a series of slats cut in a curved form to fit the member. Some splints are made of a series of slats bound together with cords in such a manner that the splint can be tightened or loosened as the surgeon sees fit during the healing process. In some cases where necessary the surgeon will remove a piece of bone from an arm or leg and insert a segment of animal bone, usually that of a sheep, or preferably a dog. Such bone transplants usually are successful.

Cauterization accompanies practically all operations, being used to arrest hemorrhage. Hot knives are often used in making surgical incisions. Several forms of cauterizing iron are used, although any convenient piece of iron may be employed, often by helpful individuals who are not surgeons. Heat is applied to various conditions such as abscesses, splenic disorders and rheumatism where the arresting of blood loss is not involved.

Berber surgeons do not perform Caesarian section, although on occasion embryotomy. Some surgeons are renowned for their ability to remove a film over the eyes.

Dentistry is practically non-existent except for the occasional extraction of teeth, which is done by jewelers because their equipment includes types of pliers and forceps that may be used in removing teeth. Bloodletting is quite frequent, often being done by laymen rather than surgeons. It usually involves making six incisions on the patient's neck, after which a bleeding cup is applied which is sucked at the tip in order to create a vacuum that promotes the flow of blood. Often drinking coffee or eating a lemon is used to reduce the feeling of exhaustion and weakness that results from the loss of blood. Bleeding on the crown of the head is considered a useful treatment for jaundice, and rheumatism is treated by bleeding or tattooing (Hilton-Simpson 1922: 78).

An impressive feature of aboriginal Berber surgery is the large number of instruments at the surgeon's disposal. Often several forms are available for a particular use. The larger instruments are of iron with wooden handles while the smaller ones are sometimes of brass or copper. By Western surgical standards these instruments appear quite crude, but their specialization and variety, achieved probably for the most part without European influence, is noteworthy. Instruments were designed for particular surgical requirements. These are specialized knives for cutting the skin, especially the scalp, in preparation for the trephine operation. Trephining drills, as previously noted, are of several types, some showing well designed features to prevent too deep penetration of the skull vault. There are a number of types of trephining saws with specialized forms, one somewhat resembling a Hey's saw occasionally used in modern Western surgery. Some of these have fine teeth; others coarse, varying from seven to three teeth per quarter inch of blade length. A variety of small instruments including retractors, elevators, hooks and forceps are used, some of the smaller ones being adapted to eye surgery. There are few needles, since suturing is rarely done, a wound being merely drawn together and bandaged. The occasionally used sutures are of silk or horse hair which are cut and removed when the wound heals.

One phase of treatment that the Berber surgeon employs was perhaps borrowed from earlier and now completely discredited European methods of dealing with edema, an abnormal increase of fluid in the body tissues. This accumulation of body fluids, that was in earlier terminology called dropsy, apparently was common in aboriginal North Africa. The native doctor's regimen of treatment is as follows: The patient's flesh is raised n folds, and strips of cotton cloth, none too clean, are soaked in a chemical consisting of copper acetate and honey. These are thrust through holes in the flesh created by inserting a red hot pointed instrument. These cloth strips, or setons, are left hanging outside the wound until they are pulled out to release the fluid accumulated in the wound area. The number of setons varies from three to six. Some are not removed but are left to come out as the skin around them deteriorates and the setons come away (Hilton-Simpson 1922: 57-58).

Minor Operations

An aspect of tissue manipulation, that by loose interpretation may be called a form of minor surgery, includes the various forms of slashing, ear piercing, lip piercing, tattooing and tooth removal or filing that have been done for either aesthetic or symbolic reasons not only in Africa but in many other parts of the world at various times in the history of culture. Some of these manipulations that are now secular and are done for beautification in terms of the cultural edicts of the group, may be derivatives of former practices that were involved with social symbolisms or supernatural figurations.

The women of the Wayo of Nyasaland have their upper lips pierced and the openings enlarged until wooden discs up to two inches in diameter are inserted. Both men and women of the Lango of Uganda are scarified in a pattern which radiates from the breast bone to the shoulders and upper arms. A bent needle or thorn is used to raise the flesh and the raised portion is cut off after which a mixture of sesame oil and red chalk is rubbed into the wound.

One form of body mutilation practiced in aboriginal Africa as well as in most other parts of the world, including even modern Europe and America, is the piercing and enlarging of the ear lobe. The people of Zanzibar pierce the ears, enlarge the opening and insert jewels, but if a person is not sufficiently affluent to afford impressive gems, the opening is further enlarged and a wooden disc about the size of a checkerman is inserted. It has been proposed that the round discs introduced into the ears may be a surviving symbol of sun worship (Harrison 1873: 198).

The chipping, filing and knocking out of teeth is quite common in Africa as a symbolic feature of initiation. Some peoples, including the Sara and Madi of central Africa and the Masai of East Africa, remove the lower central incisor teeth. The Batonga of Central Africa, on the other hand, knock out the upper front teeth. The Lango of Uganda remove the central incisors at the age of thirteen and believe that if this is not done the child will not grow to maturity. Some, such as the Yao and Makua of Central Africa, file the teeth to saw-like points. Several styles of notching the incisor teeth and filing them to points are practiced in different geographical areas (Jhering 1882: 232-237; Brabant et al. 1958: 354). An unusual form of dental filing has been noted among the Bakiga of Uganda. This involves the filing of the mesial surfaces of the upper central incisors in order to create a v-shaped diastema between the teeth. This occurs more commonly in females than in males to a ratio of nearly two to one, and is not seen among juveniles and younger children.

Early Arabian Surgery

Early Arabian surgery, like that of pre-Hippocratic surgery in Greece, is shrouded by considerable mystery. There are few documents that indicate early medical practices and such traditions as there were are not revealed in early Arabic literature. One Arabic document that reviews many customs of early Islamic times gives a little information in regard to healing methods of prior periods. This book is mainly concerned with the spiritual consolation of the sick, the evil eye, talismans and amulets, and protective prayers and formulas. There are but three types of treatment mentioned: the administration of honey, cupping and cauterization, the latter to be used sparingly. As a styptic agent the ashes of burnt matting are mentioned. The diseases cited are headache, migraine, ophthalmia, leprosy, pleurisy, pestilence and fever (Browne 1962: 12). The state of medical knowledge during this earlier period was obviously quite elementary.

As late as the tenth century A.D., Avicenna, the "Prince of Physicians" of the Arabian world (A.D. 980-1037), in his *Canon* alludes to surgery as a "manual art" and states that it is beyond the dignity of a surgeon to practice it beyond the use of the cautery and caustics (Campbell 1926: 81). Slightly earlier, Rhazes, the first great Moslem physician, defined surgery as "the art of binding up broken bones" and "dealing with wounds and ulcers" (Thorndike 1932: v. 1, 668). Albucasis of the tenth and early eleventh centuries A.D. produced a comprehensive work on surgery but it is deficient because of his lack of anatomical knowledge based on dissection, and the Moslem edict against the reproduction of the human body in any graphic or sculptural form. He did, however, illustrate and describe a considerable number of surgical instruments and a number of operations.

India: The Survival of Ear Piercing and Repair

In ancient times surgery reached a high development in India but, because of religious interdictions against dissection and an aversion to disease and blood, surgery has had no significant role in more recent traditional Indian medicine. A few minor operations have continued into the present, however, that go back to an earlier state of the surgeon's art. One of these is ear piercing, that invovles a degree of skill and an understanding of tissue growth and repair. This was observed as practiced by the Mavar tribes as follows:

This was done in infancy usually at around one month of age. The ear lobe was pierced with a needle and a cotton ligature was inserted. A knot was tied at both ends. When this was removed a straw was inserted, and after three or four days a larger piece was substituted. Finally a piece of dry pith was introduced. This was moistened with water which caused it to swell, enlarging the hole. After a fortnight pieces of cloth steeped in salt and water, and ultimately castor oil, were inserted. After one month lead or brass weights were used and these were increased in heaviness until the lower margins of both ears reached the shoulders. At puberty brass or gold replaced the earlier inserts in the ear openings and often holes were made in the upper margins of the ears and jewels inserted. At times the heavy weight of the ornaments caused the ear lobes to be torn, destroying the hole. This was considered a disgrace and a surgeon was sought who, in an ancient traditional operation, stitched the lobe together and prepared it for regrowth (Shortt 1867-8-9: 206-207).

Tibet

The surgical practices of the Tibetans, such as they are, give us some impression of the primitive Asian concepts and methods in this field as they are reported late in the last century:

Surgery is largely a layman's undertaking, although there are doctors who use some therapeutic techniques along with shamanistic performances and boasts of expertise. Some ability in the reduction of dislocations is demonstrated and fractures are reduced although apposition is often poor and deformities have resulted. There has been some use of wood splints although wood is scarce in many areas and heavy bandages are used. Hemostasis is attempted through tying a wet rag over a wound. The Tibetan surgeon occasionally performs amputations after a severe injury, not by sawing the bone but by roughly cutting the arm or leg at the place of a fracture with a knife or dagger. Scarification followed by cupping is used for rheumatism and various pains and, if this is not successful, cauterization is employed. As a further resort a crude moxibustion is applied in which cones of combustible material wrapped in silk paper are ignited and set at various places on the patient's body (Landor 1898, vol. 1: 307-314). In general, Tibetan medicine and surgery is crude and more shamanistic than naturalistic, and results are commonly disastrous to the patient.

China

Traditional Chinese medicine, as practiced by most doctors, has lacked any advanced degree of surgical accomplishment. The reason was in part a stringent Confucian ethic that abhorred blood and forbade the cutting of the dead body. Dissection was only briefly permitted and in general was not allowed until it was finally legalized through a presidential mandate of November 1913 (Major 1954: 91). Chinese medicine mainly involved a fantastically elaborate diagnostic technique of examining the pulse and a treatment that included a complex and somewhat folkloristic materia medica, also moxibustion and acupuncture.

Acupuncture required the piercing of the flesh at specified points with fine needles, of which there were many types, used either hot or cold. In applying these the disturbance of tissue was so slight that their use could scarcely be considered a form of surgery. Moxibustion, which was analogous to cauterization in Western medicine and the aboriginal medicine of Africa and numerous other areas, involved a heating and blistering of the flesh in various areas of the body. This was commonly done with a paper tube containing dried leaves of *Artemesia* or some other herbs, and ignited before applying it to the patient's body. Its value was that of a counterirritant.

There have been numerous allusions in literature, more or less fictional, to early Chinese doctors who could perform fantastic operations, some of which were in the category of major surgery (Lissowski 1967: 655-656). The greatest surgeon of ancient China, Huan T'uo (A.D. 199-268), is said to have offered to trephine the head of a general, Ts'ao Ts'ao, in order to relieve him of a headache, but because of this the general had him executed (Pollack and Underwood 1968: 36).

It is reported that early Chinese surgeons performed amputations and made incisions that were later sutured. It is also noted that in one case, Hoa Tho, who practiced between A.D. 220 and A.D. 230, used an anaesthetic, probably a preparation of hemp, administered by mouth (Ellis, E.S. 1946: 126).

Even though there may have been a few outstanding doctors in China who were capable in surgery, they were a minority and the major practice of medicine was based on animistic doctrine and treatment by herbs, massage, acupuncture and moxibustion. The extreme conservatism of Chinese culture inhibited experimentation and innovation and maintained all medical concepts and practices in a fixed state throughout many centuries.

Ainu

In considering Asian surgery Ainu tattooing must be mentioned because in the first place it involved bloodletting with a knife and moreover it was at times done for therapeutic purposes.

Ainu tattooing, which often involved complex patterns neatly executed, was done primarily on women and had the symbolic role of socially establishing their feminine attractiveness. Tattooing was mainly done on the hands and forearms and around the mouth. These were parts of the body normally exposed and therefore served as public symbols of the social entity of the individual. Yet some tattooing was done at times on parts of the body normally covered by clothing, the shoulders, back and upper arm. This was done as a cure for rheumatism or as a preventive against swelling and pain in a bruised area.

Ainu tattooing was carried out according to rigid rules. The operators were usually women and the subjects were usually girls on whom the operations started when they were seven to eight years old and continued until they were seventeen or eighteen. The operation began with scarring the skin and bloodletting. This has been more recently done with a razor, but in times past it seems to have been executed by an arrowpoint of obsidian. Soot was rubbed into the incisions. This soot was prepared in a very particular way. A carefully washed pan was hung from the ceilng over the fireplace and in it was placed bark of the white birch. After it was heated, a cloth was dipped in the residue and applied to the surface of the patient's body about to be scarified. This procedure varied from place to place but the essentials of a carefully executed procedure were observed (Kodama 1970: 117-124). It is also possible that the Ainu may have at times practiced trephination (Lisowski 1967: 656).

Japan

Japanese medicine was in most ways quite similar to that of China. Acupuncture was introduced from China but was somewhat elaborated by the Japanese, some 660 spots being indicated for the introduction of needles into the flesh of the patient and ten grades of needles were classified as to their length and thickness. The Japanese developed several schools of acupuncture depending on the type of needles used and the methods of applying them to the body (Joya 1968: 65). Bloodletting by leeches became quite popular from the ninth to twelfth centuries in Japan as a way of attempting to cure many disorders, particularly aches and swellings. Leeches were formerly sold in all cities, although the market for them is now confined to rural villages where the leech cure may still be a part of folk medicine.

Surgery in any developed sense was not a part of Japanese healing practice until it was introduced from Europe.

CHAPTER 4

OCEANIA AND AUSTRALIA

OCEANIA, including Australia, involves a segment of the earth's surface as large as Europe and Africa combined, yet much of it consists of the peaks of submerged mountains. It offers questions of great interest, geologically, biologically and ethnographically. The numerous islands of the South Pacific are the long standing homeland of peoples whose ways of life vary but show striking similarities notwithstanding wide separation by seas often difficult for navigation. How these aboriginal populations spread over vast distances of water is an intriguing question. Many Oceanic cultures show similarities over widely separated areas. To what degree these cultural elements were brought with them from elsewhere, were borrowed from neighbors or were independently invented but accidentally resemble the practices of other peoples can be debated endlessly.

These issues have particular relevance in the study of medical practices. Many procedures common in Oceania were also current in Asia and Africa, as well as the Americas. The question of regional invention versus diffusion from a common center or centers is quite beyond the scope of this discussion, but it is interesting to note that many medical practices of the Pacific Island peoples are quite similar to those found thousands of difficult navigational miles distant.

Bloodletting and Decorative Mutilation

In common with many other peoples in lesser and more advanced cultural development the inhabitants of Australia and many of the Pacific Islands practice bloodletting for various purposes through scarification and venesection. In Australia, Tasmania and the Loyalty Islands, and many other areas, it is felt that disease is the result of bad blood and that the pain or disorder will go away if the blood is released. In Fiji a gash is made in the skin and four bamboo slivers are inserted to expedite the flow of blood and bad air. In Sumatra the blood that has been removed is buried, since it is thought to be the cause of illness (Lillico 1940: 134).

A curious and inventive approach to the problem of bloodletting is that of the people of New Guinea, who, in one tribal practice, use a miniature bow with an arrow-like lancet to penetrate the flesh and promote a flow of blood from the patient. The bow is made of three midribs of coconut palm fibers bound together, and the bow string is of vegetable fiber about 20 cm. long. The arrow is tipped with a splinter of flint or broken glass. It is tied to the bow in order to prevent too deep penetration (Lillico 1940: 135; Sumner and Keller 1928, vol. 2: 1404). They also scarify with pieces of shell. Bleeding is used as a treatment for practically all kinds of pain, aches and inflammation. For fever scarification is done on the forehead and back.

Similar uses of scarification and bleeding are noted in many other Oceanic areas. In Ponape abscesses and rheumatism are thought to be aided by the release of blood. Any ailment that is not understood is treated by scarification and bleeding. In Australia headache is treated by making the nose bleed. Also among some Australians an inverse doctrine prevails. When a person becomes sick, a healthy individual is bled on his behalf. The blood, usually taken from the ulnar artery, is collected in a wooden trough. The blood is then applied over the patient's body with an emu feather brush (Thomas 1906: 44). This is perhaps a Stone Age antecedent of the blood donor-transfusion relationship.

Methods of bloodletting other than the more or less haphazard slashing of superficial blood vessels are sometimes used. Careful venesection is occasionally done in which a vein is located and opened with a sharp instrument. For this purpose the Ellice Islanders use a tooth of a rare species of shark that has a tapering shape.

Closely related to the more drastic forms of bloodletting are the methods of creating permanent scars with pigment discoloration commonly known as tatooing (a term used by Captain Cook among the Polynesians for puncturing skin and inserting pigment). While little blood may be released outside the body in this procedure, certainly blood vessels are punctured and blood is extravasated from its normal channels. The practice is widespread in both hemispheres. For tatooing designs in the Solomon Islands the skin is pierced with a bat's bone. The designs may include a tree, a fish, stars, lines representing a bank of clouds, chevrons symbolizing a snake, or the sun with radiating lines indicating sun's rays (Fox 1925: 184).

In New Guinea two fishbones are attached to a piece of wood and in operating this is tapped with another piece of wood. The wound is rubbed with blacking. The operation is done in stages since it is quite painful. This is a standard accompanying feature of adolescence for girls. It probably has religious significance since the Christianized Papuans stoutly avoid the practice (Held 1957: 28). Males are also tatooed, but purely for decoration. This is done on the chest and arms. There are no professional tatooers and anyone can do it. Girls sometimes tatoo each other. There are, however, some older women who are famed for their ability in performing this operation.

The eastern Papuans are all tatooed. The younger men tatoo their faces only, but some of the older men have patterns on their arms, legs and chest. The women are tatooed almost all over. The skin of the eastern Papuans is so dark that tatooing does not readily show on it (Haddon 1932: 100).

In the Torres Straits area tatooing is done as a mark of distinction for having taken a life. It also has certain medical applications. Y-shaped tatoo marks are applied to the back and neck for local pain and stiffness; triangular shaped marks are applied to the breast for palpitations of the heart (Seligmann 1902: 298).

The observed procedure for tattooing in New Guinea is as follows:

> The girl to be tattooed lay on the ground, and the operator held a special clay vessel in one hand, in which was a black fluid paste made from burnt resin; this was applied on the skin by means of a little stick. When the design was finished a thorn was held in the left hand, while in the right hand was a small stick round which strips of banana leaves were wound. The thorn was lightly tapped with the stick until the pattern had been well punctured into the

skin. (Haddon 1932: 113).

Scarification, or cicitrization, which may be thought of as a more drastic version of tattooing, involves cutting the flesh with knives and rubbing pigment into the wounds. If the healing is normal and uncomplicated the resulting striations in the skin may be slight and hardly noticeable except at close range. If, however, the wounds become infected, large welts may form creating pronounced ridges. In some areas this is done with great effort and consistency. In the Andaman Islands every boy and girl is scarified, always by a woman. The cuts are deep enough to draw blood but not deep enough to produce a continuous flow. Small flakes of quartz or glass are applied in short cuts in parallel rows. This is done in stages until the entire body is scarified. There are apparently two reasons for carrying out this procedure. One is merely the desire for personal adornment. The other is therapeutic: it is thought to be a cure for pain. For headache it is done on the forehead, for toothache on the cheek (Radcliffe-Brown 1948: 92, 185).

Many of the women in New Guinea "had a raised scar which extended from breast to breast — this is said to be made when a brother spears his first turtle or dogong; some had scars on various parts of their bodies, but these were the result of cuts made for the purpose of alleviating pain by bleeding" (Haddon 1932: 78-79).

In the Torres Straits area cicitrization is voluntary but quite general. The skin is cut with a piece of glass, and the chewed leaf of a certain plant is placed into the wound to prevent the edges from uniting. Wet clay is then placed over the area. This is done by an old man of known skill in the operation. An early observer states, "The Torres Strait Islanders are distinguished by a large complicated oval scar, only slightly raised, and of neat construction. This, which I have been told has some connection with a turtle, occupies the right shoulder, and is occasionally repeated on the left" (Haddon 1890: 366). Both men and women are scarified. For women the usual pattern has been a series of long lines across the hips; among men there has been considerable variety (Haddon 1890: 431).

Nose and ear piercing are often performed in the Oceanic area. In New Guinea the nasal septum is pierced when boys are young. The incision is made with a sharpened bone heated in a fire. The hole is kept open by means of a rolled up leaf and gradually increased in size. The nasal alae of both sexes are pierced in infancy. Ornaments in the form of bead strings, plaited fiber or claws of the cassowary are inserted.

Ear piercing is widely distributed. Early reports about Easter Island state that the natives had ear lobes that reached to their shoulders, and that the holes were large enough to insert four or five fingers. Sometimes the white down of sea birds was introduced. This was done with both sexes. In Borneo, the Admiralty Islands and the Solomons, large disks, some up to three inches in diameter, were placed in the opening (Harrison, J.P. 1873: 190, 195).

Genital Mutilation

Circumcision has been a prominent feature of ritual practice in Central and Northwestern Australia and Melanesia, but it is not compulsory in Borneo. In Polynesia it is widely practiced but not mandatory. It is normally done by pulling the penile foreskin of the male forward and cutting it off with a sharp stone flake. The operation is often but not always a part of an initiation ceremony. It may, as in Fiji, be a sacrificial rite undertaken as an effort to cure an ailing patient (Sumner and Keller 1928, vol. 4: 850).

A strange custom that occurs in Central Australia, parts of New Guinea, Fiji, Tonga and also among the Malays and the Chiams of Vietnam is *subincision*, the cutting of an opening into the urethra on the underside of the penis.* The operation can involve a small or a large orifice into the urethra and can run all the way from the glans penis to the scrotum. It causes considerable letting of blood. The incision is made with a knife fashioned from a quartz flake with a handle formed by pressing onto it the hardened sap of the Australian grass tree (Miklucho-Maclay 1882: 28). It apparently has no effect on the fecundity of the population and is essentially a symbolic act (Leach 1949, vol. 1: 235).

---

*This operation is sometimes called *introcision*, an undesirable usage since the term introcision is also applied to the intentional rupturing of the female hymen at the time of puberty. It can correctly be called artificial *hypospadias*, a term for an abnormal orifice on the underside of the penis. It has also been called colloquially "the terrible rite," and the mika operation.

There has been varied speculation as to the original reasons for performing subincisions. An early proposal was that it was a form of limited contraception, tending to reduce the efficiency of sexual intercourse, thereby controlling population numbers. This theory has no validity since most of the peoples who practice the operation do not recognize sexual activity as the cause of conception. It has also been cited as a means of bloodletting for therapeutic purposes and as a means of cleansing the urethra of undesirable organisms and substances. A more plausible theory is that subincision is a male counterpart of female menstruation that clears the male of noxious elements in the same manner that the female blood flow decontaminates the female (Montagu 1937: 204-207). The essence of this hypothesis is that subincision is a therapeutic procedure that cleanses the male body of noxious "humors" through an artificial opening that is anatomically analogous to the female vulva through which menstrual blood is evacuated.

In Tonga and Fiji the practice is essentially therapeutic. The urethra is opened and a thread is passed through so that one end hangs from the artificial opening and the other from the urinary meatus. The thread is at times drawn back and forth to create a discharge of blood. This procedure is frequently used as a treatment for tetanus (Rivers 1924: 105). The practice was perhaps a therapeutic measure in Tonga and Fiji and as it passed to Australia it became more ritualized and was performed five or six weeks after circumcision. It is regarded as equal in importance to circumcision (Spencer and Gillen 1927, vol. 1: 207-210). There is, however, some evidence that the practice entered Australia not from the east, but from the northwest regions and thence spread east and southeast (Elkin 1961: 165). The geographic origin of the trait in Australia is not clear but it is obvious that two aspects have become involved, therapeutic and ritualistic, both involving the cutting of sensitive tissue and bloodletting.

Among the Arunta and Ilpirra of northern Australia a girl of marriageable age is subjected to "female circumcision." This may be either *clitoridectomy*, the excision of the clitoris, or *nymphectomy*, the excision of parts of the labia minora, or even the labia majora (Montagu 1946: 422). This is performed with a stone knife and is an initiation rite equivalent to male subincision (Spencer and Gillen

1927, vol. 2: 472-473).

The Caroline Islanders, the Tonga people and the Loyalty Islanders practice a highly unusual trait of *monorchiectomy*, the compulsory removal of one testicle of all males in the population. The only other peoples known to practice this are the Hottentots, the Dama of the Western Sudan in Africa and some peoples of Ethiopia (Ackerknecht 1947: 35).

Oceanic peoples have applied some surgery in a healing capacity. In New Guinea boils were lanced with a bamboo knife; in Polynesia fractures were set with reasonable accuracy and bamboo cane splints were used to immobilize the area pending growth and repair of the fracture. In a number of areas fractures were set with bamboo splints. Dislocations were reduced through manipulation that was at times quite vigorous. Wounds were closed by drawing the edges together and applying a caustic substance. Sores were irrigated with warm water in which certain herbs had been cooked and the patient was set in the sun as an aid to healing. Tourniquets were known in the Loyalty Islands, in Tahiti, Samoa and Tonga. In Australia wounds and sprains were dressed with grease and leaves, and a large wound might be bound up with a piece of kangaroo skin. In fractures sometimes scarification was applied over the seat of the fracture and a piece of wood or bone was placed over it, bound with a section of wild vine. Lancing in Polynesia was done with a thorn or shark's tooth (Ellis, W. 1829, vol. 2: 277).

Trephining

The most outstanding feature of Oceanic surgery has been trephining of the skull. It has been reported in various places in a wide area of the Pacific ranging from the Bismarck archipelago near the equator to New Caledonia just slightly north of the Tropic of Capricorn, and eastward as far as the Marquesas around 145 degrees west latitude. The islands where trephining has been reported all lie within Polynesia and Melanesia; not Micronesia. In this cluster of island peoples, some have been widely separated by many miles of water. This operation, which is without doubt a delicate and difficult surgical maneuver, was carried out apparently with a considerable degree of success.

Trephining was done for several reasons. Many trephinations were apparently strictly medical, in order to relieve the effects of skull fracture or to remedy such disorders as neuralgia, vertigo, and headache. Head injuries were probably often caused by sling stones hurled in combat. The geographical distribution of the sling corresponds quite closely to that of trephination (Wolfel 1925: 15-17). Trephination was also performed for prophylactic reasons, in order to aid the individual being operated on to maintain health and longevity. It may also have been done for ritualistic reasons involved with supernatural powers and obligations toward these. Overlap of these roles may have been quite possible.

During the early part of the nineteenth century, the missionary William Ellis who traveled in Polynesia when native practices were still largely unmodified by Western contact, reports skull operations on the island of Bora-Bora. These involved removing fractured pieces of bone from the skull after battle casualties had resulted in crushed heads. He reports that the skin of the scalp was cleared away, the fractured pieces of bone removed, and that a piece of coconut shell was carefully fitted into the traumatized area, and the skin replaced. He notes that the operation was often successful (Ellis 1829, vol. 2: 277). On the island of New Britain there were sling stone wars in which stones about the size of a small hen's egg were hurled with great force at enemies in battle and these frequently caused fractures of the skull; also a flat two-edged club was used to attack an enemy with similar effect. The practitioner called in used a piece of shell or an obsidian flake to cut away loose fragments of the bone which he removed with his fingernail while his assistants held back the flaps of scalp. He "scraped, cut and picked away" the fractured fragments, leaving the brain exposed. The wound was bandaged with strips of banana stalk about four inches wide. The silky inner surface of these was slightly astringent and non-absorbent, allowing drainage. This bandage was renewed from time to time, and after two to three weeks the patient usually was well recovered. Death was estimated in about 20 percent of the cases, although death could often have been the result of the original trauma rather than the operation.

Samuel Ella, a missionary who had lived for some time on the island of Uvea in the Loyalty group, reports a similar operation.

The scalp is opened with a T or cross shaped incision and the cranium is scraped with a piece of glass until the dura mater is exposed. He notes that sometimes the pia mater is inadvertently penetrated, causing death. He observes that this type of trephination is also used as a remedy for headache, neuralgia and vertigo. He adds that an attempted cure for rheumatism is to lay bare the tibia or ulna and scrape the bone with a piece of glass. He reports that this curing measure was invariably unsuccessful (Ella 1874: 50-51).

There may be a question as to whether all of the cases such as those just described should be called trephinations in the strict sense where they were merely the removal of bone fragments. Often, however, the terms "scraped, cut and picked away" are used which would seem to indicate that a purposeful opening was created, in other words, a true trephination. It would appear obvious that where the operation is performed as a cure for epilepsy or neuralgia, or as a prophylactic measure where there is no head injury, it is a true trephination.

The motives for performing trephinations differ considerably from island to island as reported by early observers in the South Seas. Causes assigned by the people of several islands are as follows:

New Britain: Trephining is done only as a means of dealing with combat incurred fractures.

New Ireland: The operation is performed to treat skull fractures and also as a cure for headaches, epilepsy and insanity. Children are trephined as a prophylactic measure against ill health.

The Gazelle Peninsula: The main purpose is surgical. However, its success depends on magical interventions.

Tahiti: The purpose is purely surgical.

Loyalty Islands: The purpose is both surgical and magical. It is used to treat headache and vertigo following a blow on the head.

Mortality following a trephine operation in the South Seas has been variously estimated. One early observer reports that about fifty percent of the trephined patients died. Other reports are much more favorable. A number of skulls show successive multiple trephinations, one with eight openings in a skull from New Ireland (Margetts 1967: 676-676). These would seem to justify the belief that patients quite often survived the operation.

Amputation

The only form of amputation generally practiced in the South Seas has been the cutting off of finger joints. This has been done for a number of reasons. Interviews with native informants queried as to the reason for such amputations revealed the following:

In New Guinea: The main reason is mourning of a death. Also a cure for illness was cited, as well as purely folkloristic explanations.

In Melanesia: The mourning of a death is cited, but often no explanation is offered.

In Polynesia: The mourning of a death is the main reason, although it is also done as a cure for sickness or as a punishment. Also noted is a means of promoting success in war.

Australia: It is done to promote success in fishing: "in order to wind the fishing line better around the hand." Other explanations are that it is done in connection with betrothal and marriage, with the initiation of girls, that it is a distinguishing mark, and that it is done "in order to find yams easier." Frequently no explanation seems available (Soderstrom 1938: 40).

Normally the terminal joint of the index finger of the left hand is removed. This is often done at an early age through being bitten off by the mother. If it is done on an older individual a cobweb is tightly tied around the joint which stifles the circulation and leads to necrosis and the eventual disintegration of the joint (Spencer 1914: 10).

In general it may be noted that Oceanic surgery varies from none or the most rudimentary to the complex manipulation involved in trephining. While many of the South Sea Island natives must have had access to only the most elementary techniques of healing and little effective surgery, some of these people for various reasons were subjects of skull trephining that requires skill, patience and a certain degree of understanding of tissue characteristics. How this operation came to be employed in widely separated locations is difficult to explain. It is truly remarkable that Polynesian and Melanesian Islanders were able to achieve efficiency in this operation without appreciable surgical experience in other tissue manipulations and without the use of metals that could have furthered the making of knives, saws and other instruments.

CHAPTER 5

NORTH AND SOUTH AMERICA

THE ABORIGINAL populations of North and South America include many peoples of many cultures. In view of the fact that these peoples have lived in a variety of environments, faced varying problems of survival, and have had many contacts with peaceful and belligerent neighboring groups, it is not surprising that their medical practices have varied considerably from place to place.

Surgery, as a part of healing technology, developed apart from healing methods through medication. Medication techniques were widely used by aboriginal peoples through employing herbs and other natural ingredients that they found through experience to have had a healing effect, or were believed through their magical or folkloristic interpretation to have curing properties. Surgery, as a healing technique, involves at least some degree of understanding of human anatomy in the areas involved, along with an operative technique that depends in part on the inventive insight of the operators and also in part on the availability of materials and a knowledge of working them that could result in the making of suitable instruments for surgical use. Such peoples as the Melanesians and some of the Polynesians achieved marked success in certain forms of surgery through the use of shells and sharks' teeth, yet the most marked successes in surgery have usually occurred where metal instruments could be produced. An exception may have occurred with the early Peruvians, who were expert trephiners of the skull with stone age equipment, but in their later history used copper or bronze knives.

Trephining

Aboriginal surgery in the New World reached its greatest frequency and presumably its greatest efficiency in the Highlands of Peru. There the trephining operation on the skull was often done with confidence and usually with success. This operation was done occasionally in other parts of the Americas but nowhere to the varied degree and to the same extent that it was done in Peru and Bolivia.

The evidence for ancient aboriginal trephining in South America consists of a large number of skulls found in burial sites that have identifiable trephine openings. The total number of such skulls found in South America probably exceeds the number of trephined skulls recovered in the rest of the world. Many of these skulls are in good state of preservation, and have been carefully maintained in museum collections. A number of systematic studies have been made of these specimens. They have been reviewed in regard to age at the time of death, sex, the method used for opening the skull, possible indications of injuries that could have been the reason for the operation, and pathological conditions that might throw light on the state of health of the subject. Attention has been given to evidences of survival after the operation in the form of bone healing and repair. Such studies have been aimed at determining the role that the trephine operation may have had in the medical and supernatural phases of the aboriginal American culture. Most of these skulls are those of persons who died before the European explorers reached the region, although some date from the early post-Columbian period and some may be of later origin since in remote areas the operation may have been performed in recent times.

The possible ways by which the skull was opened by the Peruvians were scraping, cutting, sawing and drilling or punching. Each method had its advantages and hazards. Scraping is slow and of necessity covers a much wider area than the region of the proposed perforation. Cutting can be well controlled in regard to the shape and size of the desired opening and can follow the curvilinear surface of the skull, making it less likely to penetrate the dura mater of the brain than is the case with other methods. Its main disadvantage is that it requires a sharp instrument that will hold its edge under use.

Sawing requires a less refined instrument but has the disadvan-

tage of working only in straight lines creating grooves that are difficult to control in depth on a curved surface. It was undoubtedly the
fastest way of removing a bone segment from the skull vault. Drilling was probably the least satisfactory of the four methods since it
was slow, requiring a number of drilled holes, in an oval or a circle,
that were joined by cutting in order to release a more or less round
bone segment.* This method was hazardous since each drilling had
the possibility of going too far through the inner table and penetrating the brain coverings (Stewart 1957: 482). This method was rarely
used by Peruvian surgeons probably for a good reason.

Trephining by creating a series of punched holes is described by
Tello. A skull of the Yauyos in Peru shows an attempt at trephining
by punching a series of holes in a circle around the trephine area
with the planned cutting through of the divisions between the openings. Apparently the holes were not drilled but punched through the
outer table with a copper rod. The operation was not completed,
some of the bone substance planned for removal still being attached
to the margins. The existing orifice, which is less than the contem-
plated opening, is around fourteen millimeters in diameter (Tello
1913: 82-83).

Romero illustrates a skull from Monte Alban, Oaxaca, Mexico
that shows the very unusual use of a tubular trephine identical in
principle to the instrument used in Western surgery into modern
times. It was presumably a copper tube with saw teeth cut into periphery of one end and was rotated between the palms of the two
hands or with a bow (Romero 1958: 86).

Combinations of scraping and cutting or sawing are often seen in
Peruvian trephined skulls. A common operation was sawing four
grooves that eventually released a rectangular bone segment. This
method is somewhat hazardous since the operator may cut through
the inner table of the skull and into the brain coverings before he

---

*Cornejo Bouroncle illustrates a Peruvian trephined skull with sixteen drilled holes in a
more or less circular pattern (Cornejo Bouroncle 1940: 45). Moodie cites a skull
trephined by drilling in which nineteen holes were bored. These cases and other drilling
examples would have involved lengthy and tedious operations. The two cases noted show
no indication of survival after the operation, which perhaps ocurred in most if not all of
the cases of trephining by drilling because of the long time involved and the hazard of
drilling through the inner table of the skull and penetrating the coverings of the brain.

realizes the depth of his groove. Rectangular openings produced by four sawn grooves are not uncommon in Peruvian collections and this was the type used on the first Peruvian skull that became widely illustrated, one depicted in a book by E.G. Squier in 1877.*

The first detailed report on Peruvian trephining is that of Muñiz and McGee, published in 1897. This was based on a series of nineteen skulls that show trephine indications, which were drawn from a skeletal population of 1000 cases, collected from several areas of Peru (Muñiz and McGee 1897: 11-72). The majority of the specimens were determined to be those of young males presumably of military age. A series of 68 cases examined by the author[†] also from several areas of Peru yield slightly different conclusions as to sex and age. It was there found that 36, or only 60 percent were male, that 7 percent were adolescent females and that 12 percent were aged. The collections of skulls in the United States National Museum and in the Peabody Museum of Harvard University contain a number of trephined children's skulls (Stewart 1958: 481). Thus it would appear that trephinations may have been practiced on individuals of either sex and of any age although over half the subjects were male.

An important and meaningful issue is the question of to what extent trephining was employed to relieve physical damage in a traumatized area in comparison with its application where some motive was involved that left no recognizable skull damage other than the trephine wounds themselves. This is a difficult issue to resolve on the basis of evidence from the skulls alone since in many cases the actual reason for the trephining may have been a small fracture, perhaps a button of bone driven into the skull vault.

---

*Ephraim George Squier (1822-1888), an American journalist, traveler and archaeologist, wrote in 1877 a book entitled *Peru: Incidents of Travel and Exploration in the Land of the Incas*. He illustrated the frontal bone of a skull that he had acquired from a private collection and that had a small trephine opening. The skull had been found in the valley of the Yucay near Cuzco, Peru, and was unquestionably pre-Columbian. The trephine opening is a quadrangular orifice 15 mm. by 17 mm. on the left side. (It has at times been incorrectly illustrated on the right side.) The opening was made by four saw cuts that penetrated the inner table of the vault and apparently led to an easy elevation of the segment. The condition of the surrounding tissue indicates that the patient survived the operation by at least seven or eight days (Squier 1877: 457, 577-578).

[†]The 68 cases examined were collected in 1914 by Dr. Aleš Hrdlička and were a sample of the pre-Columbian skeletal population in the highlands of Peru. This collection is now maintained at the San Diego Museum of Man.

Pointed war clubs found in graves where trephined skulls have been found have been cited as the cause, also small stones hurled by slingshots. A trephine operation designed to relieve the effects of such wounds could well remove the segments of bone that contained the fracture area. The theory of pointed war clubs as the cause of such depressed fractures has been refuted on the ground that the distribution of pointed clubs is considerably wider than that of frequent trephining and that accordingly a different explanation is needed (Bushnell 1963: 64). This would tend to suggest that most military injuries were made with heavy clubs that would produce large depressions and extended fracture lines.

Some trephined skulls have been intentionally deformed, but others were not. MacCurdy reports that in a series of trephined skulls that he studied, 26 were not deformed, but that 21 were deformed by the Aymara method of binding the head to produce elongation of the skull. He feels that skull deformation has had no essential involvement with trephination (MacCurdy 1918: 393). *

Muñiz and McGee, in interpreting their skull series, noted that "(1) most of the operations were independent of cranial wounds so far as can be ascertained; (2) that most of the cranial lesions were not followed by trephining; and (3) that only wounds of great severity were followed by cranial treatment (Muñiz and McGee 1897: 67). Subsequent studies have led to different conclusions. In the series reviewed by the author it seemed clear that 13 percent of the cases showed positive relationship to an injury or a pathological state, that 37 percent were problematical, and that 49 percent showed no relation to a traumatic condition that might have led to the trephination. The lack of clear indication of a relationship between trephine openings and fractures need not be entirely meaningful since the damaged bone may have been removed as the operation progressed.

The survival of a trephine patient for an appreciable length of time is well indicated in the condition of bone tissue in the trephine

---

*In the high Andean site of Machu Pichu, 135 skulls were found but none showed trephination. Female skulls predominated (102 female; 22 male), which could perhaps be explained by the concentration of females as Virgins of the Sun in that apparently sacrosanct site, or the withdrawal of males from the same area for either combat or ceremonial duties (MaCurdy 1918: 394).

margins. In a matter of days changes usually begin in the edges of the wound which tend to obliterate the sharp striations caused by the cutting or sawing instrument or by the scraping implement (Lissowki 1867: 666). It is usually possible to assess with reasonable certainty the success of the operation in terms of the patient's survival at least for a time. There are noteworthy and dramatic evidences of survival in a number of skulls that show multiple trephinations, where the patient obviously survived one trephination to be trephined again and sometimes several times. Skulls with two or more trephine openings, some more fully healed than others, are not uncommon and as many as seven holes in Peruvian skulls have been noted (Stewart 1958: plates 1, 9 and 10). The survivorship of Peruvian trephine patients was unquestionably high, to between 70 percent and 80 percent (Rogers 1938: 331; Stewart 1958: 486).

Evidence of primitive trephining in other parts of the world often suggests a similar high degree of success. This immediately brings forth the question: How could prescientific operators with crude equipment and no aseptic provisions perform this delicate operation with such efficiency? There are three possible factors responsible.

Primarily there is evidence in many instances of technical skill on the part of the operator. In a culture where ceramics, textile weaving, stone working and metallurgy were well developed it is not surprising that manual skill and precise manipulation would have been applied to surgery. Why such ability in surgery was mainly restricted to this one operation is difficult to explain.

Another factor was undoubtedly in the conditions under which the operations were performed. Although far from aseptic, these probably were, to a considerable exent, free from many hazards of contamination and infection. The doctor probably did not attend his case immediately from another, carrying contamination on his person and instruments. The patient was not confined in a hospital where other individuals were suffering from a variety of pathological states, and the operation itself was carried out, not in an operating room where previous operations had been conducted, but rather in a well ventilated open space. All could have contributed to the healthfulness of the operating conditions.

A further factor of importance was that the patients were for the most part healthy and vigorous individuals who had survived through a severe selective process in a rugged mountainous environment.

The technique of the Peruvian trephining operation requires brief comment. As has been noted, the basic ways of opening the skull are scraping, cutting, sawing and drilling. Drilling was so rarely used that it needs little more than mention. The greatest number of Peruvian trephinations come from the central highlands where angular cutting and a combination of scraping and cutting prevailed (Stewart 1956: 302). Basically it would seem that scraping followed by either sawing or cutting was the primary method of penetrating the skull. In some cases quadrilateral saw cuts directly on the skull were used, but apparently often with unsatisfactory results. Most of the patients trephined with quadrilateral saw cuts seem to have died during or shortly after the operation (Wells 1964: 144). An important factor in the healing of bone wounds seems to be the preservation of periosteal tissue material in the wound area. Accordingly the scraping operation, which created a considerable degree of bone debris including periosteal material, would have been an advantage in bone repair (Rytel 1962: 45). Hence the type of operation that involved preliminary scraping followed by cutting would seem to have been the most efficient method.

The position of the Peruvian surgeon in relation to his patient during operating is given some probable evidence in a number of Peruvian pottery vessels. Velez Lopez illustrates one that probably shows a typical operating arrangement of the doctor and the patient. The patient is stretched out on his abdomen on a flat surface with his head raised above the level of his back. His arms are crossed over his chest and he rests on a small cushion. The surgeon is seated at the patient's side using his left hand to support and immobilize the patient's head and his right hand to manipulate an instrument, apparently a sharp pointed knife of obsidian (Velez Lopez 1940: 28).

Instruments used in Peruvian trephining were, during the earlier period, stone flakes of quartz or obsidian (Moodie 1929: 703-704). These knives were often in the form of arrow points hafted with short handles (Doig 1969: 535-536). Later, as metallurgy became more advanced, a copper or bronze knife with a curved blade was apparently used.* This was of a characteristic T-shape with a curved

---

*The Andean region was probably the first area in the New World to develop metal technology. There it was early discovered that copper alloyed with tin could produce bronze that gave durability and edge holding capacity to implements (Mason 1968: 142, 267).

blade about five inches long and with a self handle. This knife, called a *tumi*, could be conveniently held and controlled and was adapted to cutting the flesh of the scalp as well as cutting bone and removing bone fragments (Daland 1935: 556).

With time the trephine operations included smaller skull areas than in the early period (Wakefield and Dellinger 1939: 168). This could have been the result of two factors. The surgeons were no doubt becoming more efficient and managed the location of a trephine opening with more precise reference to the trauma for which the trephination was being performed. Again this change may have resulted from an increasing realization that the patient's difficulties were the result of a specific local involvement of the skull rather than a vague need to permit the escape of malicious elements.

The question most frequently asked in regard to aboriginal trephining probably is, Why was it done? Since Peru was the area of most intensive practice of this form of aboriginal surgery, skeletal materials from there should give us the best clues as to an answer. In general there are eight possible reasons for the primitive trephining of the skull. These are:

(1)   The removal of bone fragments in a depressed fracture that appears to cause disturbance in body function,

(2)   To reduce the effects of periostitis, inflammation or syphilitic lesions (Tello 1913: 76),

(3)   The reduction of intracranial pressure caused by some supposed condition other than a fracture,

(4)   To permit the escape of some entities or substances that are assumed to be the cause of the illness such as evil spirits or bad blood,

(5)   A prophylactic measure that for some mystic reason is thought to promote health and well-being during later life,

(6)   A type of ordeal, initiation rite or other ritual,

(7)   To obtain a part of a trephined skull to be used as an amulet thought to have mystic properties, and

(8)   A postmortem operation for practice in training surgeons (Wells 1964: 145), or perhaps involved with a head trophy cult (Stewart 1958: 475).

Several of these options can reasonably be discarded as far as the

Peruvians are concerned. Postmortem operations could have been made, but the high percentage of healing in the examples recovered would certainly suggest that most of the operations of which we have evidence were premortem.

The percentage of obvious cases where trephination is associated with the skull fractures would tend to throw doubt as to the likelihood that trephinations were normally used for prophylactic or ritual reasons. This would limit the possibilities to:

(a)   Naturalistic efforts to relieve the damaging effects of skull fractures, and

(b)   Mystical undertakings to remove from the body of the patient supposed malicious forces that are thought to be causing a disorder.

MacCurdy, in a number of cases recovered by an expedition sponsored by Yale University and the National Geographic Society in 1914, reported that most of the trephinations were apparently to relieve depressed fractures but that a number of traumatic areas were not followed by a surgical operation. He also noted that in only one case in his series was there an instance where an operation was apparently conducted to releve a condition that involved diseased bone (MacCurdy 1923: 260, 263).

However, as with all prescientific peoples, much of illness is mysterious, and there is a strong likelihood that any naturalistic attempt to deal with physiological phenomena often becomes involved with supernatural approaches.

A puzzling question arises as to the quality of the Peruvian operation. A cursory examination of trephined skulls in museum collections reveals that different technical grades of the operation appear to be indicated. Some show a precise and carefully managed undertaking while others appear to be crude and badly executed. This could perhaps result from two grades of surgical professionalism, one that was practiced by a trained corps of experts who conserved through personal transmission a body of knowledge and a tradition of performance, and the other that was undertaken by poorly trained individuals who were perhaps priests who assumed supernatural authority and preyed on the ignorance and gullibility of their followers to perform spectacular and often disastrous operations as demonstrations of their divine power and prestige. The results of such operations, as can be seen in the Museum collections at Cuzco, show what appears to be the irresponsible hacking away of a good portion of the patient's skull with obviously fatal results. Two grades of surgery appear to be indicated, one that resulted from a tradition of knowledge and practice and the other that developed from pretense, ignorance and incompetence.

One persisting question in regard to the occurrence of trephining in primitive cultures is, Why was this complicated and difficult operation, one that is regarded medically as exacting major surgery, attempted so often and so casually by many aboriginal peoples? A contributing thought in answer might be that prescientific peoples often thought of the head as a part of the body without specific function except as a region that might on occasion be the seat of disturbance such as headache and neuralgia. Its neurological role and sensitivity as the prime center of nervous coordination, memory and judgment was unknown to them; therefore, if the head ached why not cut into it and get out whatever was wrong?

Occasional trephine operations were directed toward the frontal sinus. This was presumably to relieve pain caused by emphysema in this cavity (Burton 1920: 324; Canelis et al. 1981: 186-189).

It has been noted that cauterization on the head may have been used by American Indians possibly to relieve aches and stress and that this could have produced lesions that have been interpreted as trephinations (Hrdlička 1939: 166-167). It can be noted that cauterization might involve the outer table of the skull over a considerable area and that this could heal, producing a condition similar to a healed trephination.

Occasionally the Peruvian surgeon placed an insert or covering over the trephine opening. This would have had two purposes, to protect the delicate brain from damage by outside contacts and to prevent herniation of the brain through the opening. Different materials were used, gourd, bone, shell, silver and gold. These were apparently useful since skulls where these coverings have been found show evidence of survival, at least for a time. Although this would seem to have been a desirable practice, it was done but rarely, however.

There is frequent speculation as to what degree the Peruvians

may have used drugs as narcotics for producing anesthesia in surgery. It has been suggested that they used coca and peyote as anes-
thetics (Bandelier 1904: 445; Vogel 1970: 163, 193, 408-409). It has
been noted that the Peruvian Indians in more recent times have
treated a wound prior to surgical manipulation with powdered
leaves that contain some 9 percent of cocaine, and that this nullifies
pain that might result from the operation (Ellis, E.S. 1946: 108). It
is further suggested that this technique of local anesthesia could well
have been used by the Peruvians in carrying out their trephining
operations, but that there is no evidence that such measures were
used in prehistoric European surgery. One proposal has been that
anesthesia was produced by injecting with an enema syringe a solu-
tion of *parica* or *cohoba* made from the seeds of the tree *Piptadenia pere-
grina* (Nordenskiöld 1930: 187). Again it has been suggested that
large quantities of chicha or corn beer may have aided in dulling the
patient's sensitivity (Doig 1969: 536). For the ancient past this is of
course speculative but since these botanicals were available and coca
is currently used by some South American Indians as a painkiller
and hunger depressant, it is hard not to believe that the resourceful
doctors of the past would have used them to quiet their patients and
make their operations more smooth running.

Although the Andean region was the area of most intensive development of head surgery in the Americas, trephined skulls have
occasionally been reported as far north as Alaska and as far south as
Chile and southern Argentina. Stewart lists seventeen cases of "puta-
tive trephining" from North America, distributed from Alaska to
southern Mexico (Stewart 1958: 478-479) (see Map 2). A number of
these are incomplete and not all have been fully studied. One of the
unusual occurrences is the discovery of two trephined female skulls
from the Tarahumara region of northern Mexico. Neither have
traumatic or pathological indications and both show full healing.
The evidence is clear that the trephining operation was within the
capability of these remote people (Lumholtz and Hrdlička 1897:
389-396). Two trephined skulls have been reported from New Mexico. One is a diseased skull with a 40 mm. by 50 mm. opening in the
frontal bone and no evidence of recovery. The other skull has a
diamond shaped opening 20 mm. in diameter in the right parietal
bone with indication of postoperative repair (Shapiro 1927: 266-

269). The method used appears to have been scraping and cutting. No relationship is indicated between the practice here and in Peru (Moodie 1930a: 908).

A trephined skull is reported from Georgia with an opening 38 mm. in diameter across the right and left parietal bones. It shows little healing (Cosgrove 1929: 353-357).

During the course of archaeological excavations in a shell-heap on the border between British Columbia and Washington in 1922, two trephined skulls were found. Both have more or less circular cut trephine openings, one on the left side of the frontal bone, the other on the right parietal. Both are of mature females. There is little healing but sufficient to indicate that the operations were performed during life (Smith, H.I. 1924: 447-452).

A number of reported cases of trephining in the Americas are clouded with some doubt as to the interpretation of the wound as a trephination in the strictest sense. An example is from an old Indian burial in southern Connecticut. It was reported as a "deliberate antemortem trephination of the scraping type." The diagnosis has been proposed, however, that the opening may be the result of a cyst or tumor (Powell 1970: 732-734). Whether this, along with several others in North America, were actually trephinations is open to question.

Some seven skulls have been reported from Michigan, mostly from the Rouge River area, that have circular cut perforations varying in diameter from 15 mm. to 20 mm. The perforations are all on the top of the skull in the middle on the sagittal suture and somewhat posterior to the bregma. None indicate healing and they are all interpreted as postmortem (Gillman 1876: 237-244). It has been proposed that these openings were made in order to suspend the skull by means of a cord presumably from some part of the house structure since it has been the practice of some Indians to retain the skulls of ancestors or slain enemies for supernatural reasons. The small percentage of these perforated skulls in proportion to the numbers of those not so treated that have been recovered in the Michigan area would tend to cast some doubt as to this interpretation, however.

Among the American Indians surgery reached its most advanced development among the peoples of the high Andes in South America; yet it was practiced in a lesser way by various others in

South America and in North America. Many forms of minor surgery were understood and used in various areas.

Amputation and Minor Surgery

Amputation in many areas was carefully avoided for certain magico-religious reasons. Some peoples, however, were quite willing to amputate members of the body. A case is mentioned among the Chippewa in which a man whose legs and feet were frozen when he was a boy had both his legs amputated. This was done with a common knife and the only dressing was of bark. The healing, however, had been complete (Densmore 1928: 333-334). The Patagonians of southern Argentina are reported frequently to have practiced amputation and to have gained anatomical knowledge from so doing (Corlett 1935: 242). The Assiniboin and Crows of North America have often amputated fingers as a form of mourning sacrifice. This is done with a sharp knife or with a tomahawk which was struck after the finger was placed on a block. Usually the first and second joints are sacrificed but with men the thumb and middle finger on the left hand and the thumb and two forefingers of the right hand are preserved for the use of a bow or rifle (Denig 1930: 427). Young Sioux warriors cut off the little fingers of the left hands after the Sun Dance ritual (Bourke 1892: 485).

There is considerable evidence that the Peruvians may have, from time to time, performed amputations. A number of pottery vessels depict stumps of extremities that appear to be the result of amputations, although there is the possibility that some of these may have resulted from pathological conditions such as lepra, syphilis or leishmaniasis rather than surgical amputations (Ackerknecht 1947: 31). There is considerable evidence, however, from the sculptural treatment of Peruvian pots, that facial features representing destructive lesions of the *uta* disease often also show indications of surgical manipulation probably in treatment (Salaman 1939: 115-116). Also it is important to note that certain of these pots represent individuals who have had parts of arms and legs amputated and have been fitted with wooden protective caps that have been found in their graves. A mummy was found with an amputated leg and attached to it a wooden prosthesis that showed marks of wear in walking. Such evidences tend to indicate that amputation was probably a well planned operation in Peruvian surgical practice.

Amputation for the identification and retention of criminals is reported for several North American areas. The Senecas are said to have amputated a portion of the feet of prisoners, cutting away "half of the foot" and wrapping skin over the stump, apparently with success in healing since the prisoners so mutilated were said to have been able to walk, but with some difficulty, and to have left characteristic footprints that made them easy to track in their efforts to escape (Packard 1963, vol. 1: 20). This operation has been further described as "cutting off half of their feet lengthwise so that they would not be able to run away" (Swanton 1928: 705).

Possible cases of amputation have included a hand in a late Hopewell culture site of Illinois (500 B.C.-500 A.C.) and a hand of a Mayan skeleton from Guatemala (Steinbock 1976: 36-38). An amputation of a humerus from Peru suggests that the operation may have been performed there in pre-Columbian times (Rogers 1973). This example is a partial humerus from Lupo, Peru, near Huarochiri. The bone has clearly had the lower portion cut off and the remaining part is 147 mm. long (a normal complete humerus of a Peruvian female would be around 270 mm. long). There is no indication of pathology or prior surgery. The bone is that of a young female who survived the operation by a number of years.

The Peruvians also apparently amputated parts of the nose and lips, as well as the leg (Moodie 1920a: 216, 227).

The amputation of fingers and at times toes was a frequent mourning obligation for South American women and at times also men. It has been reported that among the tribes of the Paraná River delta in southern Argentina women have commonly been seen with no outer joints of the fingers remaining and that some men have only thumbs left because of this practice (Metraux 1947: 30).

Lancing, scarification and bloodletting were practiced by a number of American Indians, but a practice of the Chippewa is worthy of special mention. An instrument consisting of a number of needles fitted into a wood handle was used to introduce medicine under the skin. A description of the procedure is as follows:

An instrument for applying a medicine beneath the skin consisted of several needles fastened at the end of a wooden handle. This was used in treating "dizzy headache," neuralgia, or rheumatism in any part of the body. In giving the treatment the medicine was "worked in" with the needles. If only a small part were to be "gone over" it was customary to hold a knife in the left hand and to use the blade as a guide for the needles. These were "worked up and down" close to the blade, "which kept the medicine from spreading." The remedy used most often in this manner was made as follows: Hazel stalks or cedar wood was burned to a charcoal and a small quantity of the charcoal (or ash) was mixed with an equal quantity of the dried gall of a bear. It was mixed well and placed in a birch-bark dish. When used it was moistened a little with water and stirred, after which a little was taken on the blade at the end of the wooden instrument and laid on the affected part. It was then "worked in" with the needles. The dark spots seen on the temples of many Indians are left by the charcoal in this medicine. A remedy for rheumatism was applied in a similar manner. The plant was identified as *Trillium grandiflorum* (Miehx.) Salisb., and it was used in the form of a decoction. (Densmore 1928: 333).

This is clearly an example of prescientific hypodermic injection for medical purposes and along with it unplanned tattooing.

Bloodletting was widely practiced in South America in order to enhance the strength of the arms and legs. It was done prior to many kinds of activity that required strength and muscular control. It was felt that weakness resulted from the presence of malicious elements in the blood and that to release these through bleeding aided the individual in his physical efforts. With the Incas to relieve sickness this was done with a sharp stone point on the end of a stick; among the Amazon tribes it was done with a small arrow with a crystal point that was shot into the patient with a miniature bow (Karsten 1926: 156-159).

Occasional instances of purposeful and well managed incision are reported for North American Indians. An operation by a Zuñi Indian doctor in order to drain a breast abscess is noted where the doctor anesthetized the patient with Jimson weed, *Datura stramonium*, after which he opened the patient's breast with a stone knife, explored the area with his finger and removed the accumulated pus with apparently little distress on the part of the patient (Stone 1962: 86).

Although rare, the suturing of wounds was sometimes done with considerable efficiency. The Guiana Indians are reported to have done this with the use of ants. The large South American leaf cutting ants were placed so that they grasped the two margins of a wound with their jaws and held these in place, after which the ants' heads were severed from the bodies (Majno 1975: 304).

The Point Barrow Eskimo performed some types of very crude surgery. Suffering patients at times scarified their own backs to relieve rheumatism and their scalps to relieve headache. One individual lost the last joint of his forefinger as a result of an exploding cartridge with a stump of bone protruding. An Indian doctor cut the stump off with a chisel (Murdoch 1892: 423).

Among the Plains Indians of North America the amputation of fingers and hands of enemies seems to have been an important symbolic and ceremonial procedure. Bourke reports that after a raid on a Cheyenne village the recovered artifacts, presumably valuable property, included necklaces of amputated fingers and a bag filled with the right hands of papooses of the Shoshoni, deadly enemies of the Cheyenne (Bourke 1892: 481). How the amputations were performed is not known, but it may well be assumed that the method was a crude chopping.

A difficult and unusual operation is reported for the Loucheux Indians of Canada. A white man who suffered from a fractured patella as a result of a logging accident was operated on by an Indian woman. In that tribe all of the surgery is done by women. The operator made three cuts on the underside of the knee and pulled the skin back to expose the patella. She used an obsidian flake, freshly chipped from a block of the stone. On being interrogated as to why they used obsidian flakes rather than the sharp steel knives that they had, the reply was that the freshly chipped stone was cleaner than the steel. Pegs of caribou bone were prepared and pressed into the ligaments above and below the fractured segments. Then a piece of caribou sinew, drawn out to create a firm cord, was wound back and forth between the pegs and used to draw the separated elements together. The flap of skin was replaced and bound with thongs. No suturing was used. The operation required between two and three hours. After several months of convalescence and inactivity the patient returned to a city where he was examined and given further postoperative care. The patella appeared to be fully healed without infection (Graham 1930: 234-235).

Of the aboriginal peoples of the North American continent at the time of the first European exploration, the Aztecs were the most culturally advanced. They had developed a politically complex state and had achieved a high level of technology equalling in many ways that of Europe of the same chronological period. Their status in regard to medicine, and in particular surgery, is worth noting in particular since their achievements, although not strictly scientific, were those of a literate people with a capacity for meticulous observation and with well established cultural traditions.

Aztec knowledge of human anatomy was apparently considerable, although it seems not to have been used to a great extent in the interpretation of body disorders and healing ministrations. Vocabularies of terms in the Nahuatl language of the Aztecs include words for many parts of the body. The most numerous and specific are those for the extremities and their associated structures. Next in order of richness in vocabulary are terms for the trunk, head, integument, reproductive apparatus, bones, organs of sensation, and internal structures. A knowledge of visceral anatomy is indicated by terms for the heart, stomach, intestines, liver, kidneys, bladder and other internal body details (Sahagún 1961: 95-138; Rogers and Anderson 1966: 71-73; Austin 1980: vol. 1). The degree of development in Aztec medicine is reflected in their categories of practitioners which include doctors who prescribed medicines to be taken internally or applied to the skin; surgeons who performed operations that involved cutting of the skin; phlebotomists or bloodletters; pharmacists who prepared and administered remedies, largely herbal; and specialists who dealt in particular with wounds, fractures and tumors.

Since the Aztec state was in a continuous condition of hostility with many other peoples within their range of contacts, which was wide in MesoAmerica, the practice of surgery seems quite understandably to have been mainly involved with the handling of military casualties. Accordingly the treatment of wounds and fractures appears to have been their most effective area of medical practice. They sutured with hair and were able to reduce fractures with skill.

In dealing with fractures they applied a mixture of resin with powdered seeds of *Datura stramonium*, over which they laid bird feathers and over these slats were bound in order to hold the bone segments in place (Clavijero 1975: 184). If healing did not progress satisfactorily the broken bones were scraped and reset (Bancroft 1883: 600).

Along with many other American Indians they resorted frequently to bloodletting which they accomplished with obsidian knives, porcupine quills and maguey thorns.

Trephination seems not to have been an Aztec specialty. However, according to the Florentine Codex of Sahagún, our most reliable and detailed contemporary observer of Aztec culture, a broken skull is "joined with a bone awl, is covered with maguey sap, or a grated green maguey leaf is applied" (Sahagún 1961: 141). The meaning of this statement is open to some speculation. Apparently the term interpreted as "bone awl" may also be construed as a "piece of bone" and may well mean that the surgeon's role was to bring together the broken fragments of the skull vault and restore these to their suitable anatomical relationship, after which they were given proper medication.* While this was perhaps not trephination it probably served the same purpose that trephination provided in some cultures, namely the management of a fractured skull so that the bone fragments did not impinge on the brain covering.

The Aztecs were apparently quite capable in dealing with minor eye operations. The Florentine Codex includes the statement: "Fleshy growth over the eyes: as a cure the growth over the eye is raised up with a maguey thorn; it is cut" (Sahagún 1961: 144). This is most probably an operation for pterygium that perhaps resulted from ultraviolet radiation in a polution free high altitude environment.

Dental mutilation was extensively practiced in the New World apparently for a variety of reasons. The most frequent purpose was probably for a decoration but it was also done as a symbol of initiation, to demonstrate mourning and to make the human teeth resemble in shape those of an animal that perhaps had totemic significance (Comas 1966: 374-376). Inlays of turquoise, jadeite, pyrite and other substances were sometimes inserted into round drilled holes.

---

*Arthur J.O. Anderson 1984: personal communication.

Considerable attention has been given to the nature of the cement used to hold the inlays and overlays in place, since these appear to have been highly durable. Spectrographic analyses have revealed that a number of elements were present in the cement, but that calcium and phosphorus were in high perecentage, with perhaps the addition of silicon. Some organic substances may also have been used. Numerous styles of filing, drilling and inlaying were developed and these varied with the region and culture period (Romero 1958). Gold inlays and overlays were used in Ecuador. In one case a skull with an implanted tooth with a gold inlay was discovered (Saville 1913: 381).

In Mexico twenty-four types of tooth mutilation have been identified and practically all have been done on postadolescent individuals and all are premortem (Borbolla 1940).

It is difficult to summarize the aboriginal surgery of the New World since American Indian surgical techniques in at least some groups seem to have included practically all the surgical devices known in the Old World prior to Hippocratic times, and perhaps more. A concise summary might be that the New World aborigines in some of their numerous tribal areas were apparently as inventive and efficient in surgery as any other prescientific peoples in history. In some groups medical knowledge and skill equaled or surpassed the state of the healing arts in Europe at the beginning of the sixteenth century, when Europeans first explored the Americas.

The foregoing discussion is directed toward the question, At what time in history and under what circumstances did humans arrive at the idea that they could heal disorders, beautify the body, socially categorize an individual or punish an offender by tampering with human flesh through cutting, burning, scarring or piercing? That such efforts were universal suggests that the urge toward flesh manipulation parallels the entire history of culture. The fact that in one area such impulses became the basis of scientific surgery was primarily the result of Greek culture that fostered the orderly recording of observations, seeking truth through experiment, and the progressive extraction of magic and mysticism from healing disciplines. Throughout the course of varied advancements and recessions medicine progressed from primitive empiricism to a modern science. Not all aspects of surgery, however, have been dedicated to curing illness and healing injuries. A few of these have survived in wide distribution, such as tattooing and ear piercing. The general urge toward tissue manipulation may be older than the healing arts and medical surgery may perhaps be looked upon as the fortunate by-product of an ancient urge to maneuver and tamper with human flesh for varied casual reasons.

GLOSSARY

ACUPUNCTURE. Various attempted healing efforts that employ puncturing the skin with needles which are manually vibrated by the operator, or in more recent practice are activated by electricity. It is based on a theory of nerve physiology that embraces a complex of nerve channels throughout the body that can be tapped by puncturing the skin at specific points at which the nerve system is specifically sensitive and related to other areas.

AMULET. A device worn or carried to ward off evil forces. Its efficacy may reside in either its substance or its shape.

BOUGIE. An instrument for exploring and dilating canals. It may be hollow or solid, but is usually flexible.

BRONZE AGE. The period in prehistoric archaeology following the Neolithic or New Stone Age and before the Iron Age. It ranged from 3,500 B.C. to 750 B.C., varying in different areas. It was characterized by the alloying of copper with tin in the making of implements, and the rarity of tin brought about more extensive travel and conquests than had been required when copper was the sole metal used.

CAESARIAN SECTION. The delivery of a fetus by an incision into the uterus, usually through the abdominal wall. It is done when there are risks to the baby from natural childbirth such as breech presentation that cannot be turned or when it is too large to pass through the birth canal. Julius Caesar was said to have been delivered in this manner.

CARIES, DENTAL. The localized decay and disintegration of

tooth enamel, dentine and often also the cementum.

CASTRATION. The removal of the sex glands, the testes or ovaries. Castration of the male is termed orchidectomy; of the female oophorectomy or ovariectomy.

CAUTERIZATION. Burning and the killing of tissue through the application of a hot iron or a corrosive substance. It has been used to arrest the flow of blood, to sterilize an area and at times merely as a counterirritant.

CICATRIX (pl. CICATRICES). A scar formed by new tissue produced in the healing of a wound. Scars for body ornamentation are formed by raising the skin and cutting with a knife. Infection causes the scars to become larger and more obvious.

CIRCUMCISION, FEMALE. The excision of the clitoris and portions of the labia minora and at times also the labia majora. Also called CLITORIDOTOMY.

CLITORIDOTOMY. See CIRCUMCISION, FEMALE.

COCA. Leaves of the South American plant *Eurythroxylon coca*, resembling tea in appearance. The source of cocaine. A stimulant and narcotic.

CROCHET. An obstetrical instrument in the form of a pointed hook.

CURRETAGE. Scraping to remove growths or other matter from the walls of a body cavity. The spoon-like instrument used for this is a CURETTE.

DEBRIDEMENT. The removal of dead tissue and foreign matter in the area of a wound.

DIPLOË. The spongy tissue between the two tables of cranial bones that contain red bone marrow.

DURA MATER. The fibrous covering of the brain.

EDEMA. Swelling as a result of excessive fluid in the intercellular spaces of the body tissue. DROPSY is an obsolete term for generalized edema.

ELEVATOR. An instrument for lifting a depressed part of bone or other tissue. A common form has a slightly curved shallow spoon-like blade.

EMBRYOCTONY. The destruction of the embryo or fetus.

EMPIRICAL. Based on observation and experience without regard to science or the knowledge of principles.

FIRE DRILL. A device used to kindle fires consisting of a shaft rotated either between the palms of the hands or by means of a bow. Friction between the end of the shaft and a depression in the hearth plate generates sufficient heat to ignite tinder and cauterize flesh.

GIGLI SAW. A saw for cutting bone consisting of a steel wire with sharp teeth cut along its length. It is held and operated by handles at the two ends.

GLOSS. An explanation usually in the form of a marginal note that explains terms or statements in the text of a document.

HEMOSTATIC. A drug or manipulation that tends to arrest hemorrhage.

HIPPOCRATIC CORPUS. A series of Greek documents that summarize the principles of Hippocratic medicine. It is doubtful that all or any were written by Hippocrates himself since they vary in style and are not all consistent in content.

INFIBULATION. The closure either by stitching or the application of a binding ring or clasp on the male prepuce or the labia majora of the female in order to prevent sexual union.

INTROCISION. The intentional rupture of the female hymen at the time of puberty. The term is sometimes applied to SUBINCISION (q.v.).

IRON AGE. The archaeological phase from around 1000 B.C. to the beginning of the Christian era. It is marked by a change in technology resulting from the discovery of iron smelting that brought an improvement over the copper and bronze previously employed.

JIMSON WEED. *Datura stramonium*, a plant with white or violet funnel-shaped flowers with poisonous and narcotic properties.

LITHOTOMY. The incision of an organ for the removal of a stone or calculus.

MEDICINE MAN. A practitioner in aboriginal societies who is believed to have knowledge and supernatural expertise capable of healing and dealing with all types of human crises. He may or may not combine a measure of naturalistic healing technique with his mystical ministrations.

MESIAL. A term of anatomical reference meaning toward the middle plane of the body. Applied to teeth referring to the surface toward the middle of the dental arch.

MONORCHIECTOMY. The excision of one of the two male testes.

MOXIBUSTION. The use of a burnable material in a convenient form ignited to apply heat to a specific area of the body. A somewhat controlled and refined form of cauterization.

NEOLITHIC. The New Stone Age — marked by the making of polished stone implements and the beginnings of agriculture and the extensive domestication of animals. The basic technological and social foundation of modern civilization.

NOSEPIN. A pin usually of bone, inserted through an orifice punctured in the nasal septum.

ORCHIDECTOMY. See CASTRATION.

PALEOLITHIC. The Old Stone Age: the earliest archaeological phase as designated through implement types. Paleolithic implement styles shade back into the Eolithic, a hypothetical period during which human beings first began to supplement their hands and fingers with mechanical accessories in the form of chipped stones and sharpened sticks.

PAPYRUS. A tall aquatic plant, *Cyperus papyrus*, widely grown in the Nile Valley. Strips of the plant were soaked, pressed together and dried, creating the fundamental writing material for the Egyptians, Greeks and Romans. In Egyptian archaeology "papyrus" is taken merely to mean a manuscript, because they were inscribed on papyrus surfaces.

PHLEBOTOME. A thin double edged surgical knife used in opening blood vessels.

PHLEBOTOMY. The surgical opening of a vein. Syn.: VENESECTION.

PIA MATER. The delicate innermost covering of the brain and spinal cord. It contains many blood vessels and dips into the various fissures of the brain.

PROCTOLOGY. The branch of medicine that deals with diseases of the anus, rectum and colon.

RASPATORY. An instrument used for scraping periosteum from bone. It has a blade with a beveled scraping edge.

RETRACTOR. An instrument used to pull tissues aside in order to facilitate an operation.

RHINOPLASTY. A surgical operation designed to correct the form of a nose that has been misshapen through injury, wound or congenital defect.

RONDELLE. A disk; applied anthropologically to portions of cranial bones removed from the skull by trephining.

SETON. A strand of linen or silk drawn through a wound in the skin in order to facilitate drainage.

SINCIPETAL. Related to the upper half of the skull or SINCIPUT.

SOUND. A tubular surgical instrument, often curved, used in exploring body cavities or dilating canals.

STRIGIL. An instrument with a curved blade used by the Greeks and Romans to scrape the skin after bathing or exercise.

SUBINCISION. The making of a surgical incision on the underside of the penis opening into the urethra. The opening is usually at least one inch in length.

TATTOOING. The puncturing of the skin and insertion of an indelible pigment. There are varied techniques and a great range of designs and patterns are employed. Portions of the body or the entire body may be involved.

TENACULUM. A fine pointed hook used in surgery to pick up and hold tissue.

TREPANNING. See TREPHINING.

TREPHINE. An instrument used for trephining, in the form of a tube with saw teeth cut into the periphery.

TREPHINING. The surgical removal of tissue with a trephining instrument. Most often used with reference to opening the skull by removing a segment of cranial bone.

TROCAR. A surgical instrument consisting of a pointed rod inserted in a tube, used for piercing body cavities and withdrawing fluid.

TUMI. An aboriginal Peruvian bronze knife with a half moon shaped blade and self handle.

VENESECTION. Bloodletting by opening a vein.

BIBLIOGRAPHY

Ackerknecht, Erwin H.: Contradictions in primitive surgery. Bull Hist
Med 20 (2): 184-187, 1946.
————— : Primitive surgery. Amer Anthropol 49 (1): 25-45, 1947.
————— : A short history of medicine. New York, The Ronald Press Co.,
1968.
————— : Medicine and ethnology: selected essays. Baltimore, The Johns
Hopkins Press, 1971.
Austin, Alfredo López: Medicina Náhuatl. México D.F., Univ Nac Auto
de México 1975.
————— : Cuerpo humando e ideologia; las concepciones de los antiguos
Nahuas. vol. 1. México D.F., Univ Nac Auto de Mexico, 1980.

Baas, Joh. Hermann: Outlines of the history of medicine and the medical
profession. Translated by H.E. Handerson. Huntington, New York,
Robert E. Krieger Publishing Co., 1971.
Bancroft, Hubert Howe: The Native Races vol. 2, Civilized Nations. San
Francisco, A.L. Bancroft & Company, Publishers, 1883.
Bandelier, Adolph F.: Aboriginal trephining in Bolivia. Amer Anthropol
n.s. 6: 440-446, 1904.
Bartels, Max: Die Medizin der Naturvölker: ethnologische Beiträge zur
Urgeschichte der Medicin. Leipzig, T. Greiben, 1893.
Barton, Juxon: Notes on the Kipsikis or Lumbwa tribe of Kenya Colony.
J Roy Anthropol Inst 53: 42-78, 1923.
Berdoe, Edward: The origin and growth of the healing art; a popular his-
tory of medicine in all ages and countries. London, Swan, Sonnens-
chein & Co., 1893.
Biggs, Robert: Medicine in ancient Mesopotamia. In History of Science,
an Annual Review of Literature, Research and Teaching, vol. 8, 94-

105. Cambridge, W. Heffer and Sons, Ltd., 1969.

Borbolla, D.F. Rubin de la: Types of tooth mutilation found in Mexico. Am J Phys Anthropol 26: 349-362, 1940.

Bourke, John G.: The medicine-men of the Apache. Ann Rept Bureau of Amer Ethnol 9: 443-603. Washington, Govt. Printing Office, 1892.

Brabant, Hyacinthe; Klees, Louis and Werelds, René J.: Anomalies, mutilations et tumeurs des dents humaines. Paris, Éditions Julien Prelat, 1958.

Brandon, S.G.F., ed.: A dictionary of comparative religion. New York, Charles Scribner's Sons, 1970.

Breasted, J.H.: The Edwin Smith Papyrus. 2 vols. Chicago, Univ. of Chicago Press, 1930.

Brothwell, Don: The bio-cultural background of disease. In Brothwell and Sandison, 1967, pp. 56-68.

Brothwell, D.R.: Digging up bones; the excavation, treatment and study of human skeletal remains. Third ed. Ithaca, New York, Cornell Univ. Press, 1981.

Brothwell, Don, and Sandison, A.T.: Diseases in antiquity: a study of the diseases, injuries and surgery of early populations. Springfield, Ill., Charles C Thomas, Publisher, 1967.

Browne, A.T.: Zulu medicine and medicine men. Cape Town, C. Struik, 1970.

Buck, Albert H.: The growth of medicine from the earliest times to about 1800. New Haven, Yale Univ. Press, 1917.

Burton, Frank Albert: Prehistoric trephining of the frontal sinus. Calif. State J of Med 18: 321-324, 1920.

————— : Some considerations on prehistoric aural, nasal, sinus pathology and surgery. Pub School of Amer Res, 1927.

Bushnell, G.H.S.: Ancient peoples and places; Peru. New York, Frederick A. Praeger, 1963.

Campbell, Donald: Arabian medicine and its influence on the Middle Ages. Vol. 1. London, Kegan Paul, Trench, Trubner & Co. Ltd., 1926.

Canalis, Rinaldo F.; Hemenway, William G.; Cabieses, Fernaldo; and Aragon, Roberto: Prehistoric trephining of the frontal sinus. Anns of Otology, Rhinol and Laryngol 90(2): 186-189, 1981.

Castiglioni, Arturo: A history of medicine. Translated by E.B. Krumbhaar. New York, Jason Aronson, Inc., 1975.

Chauvet, Stephen: La médecine chez les peoples primitifs (Préhistoriques et contemporaines). Paris, Libraire Maloine, 1936.

Clavijero, Francisco Javier: La medicina de los Mexicanos. In Austin, Alfredo López, 1975, 179-184.

Comas, Juan: Manual de antropología física. México, D.F., Univ Nac Auto de Mexico, 1966.

Coon, Carleton S. and Hunt, Edward E., Jr., eds.: Anthropology A to Z. New York, Grosset and Dunlap Inc., 1963.

Corlett, William Thomas: The medicine man of the American Indians and his cultural background. Springfield, Ill., and Baltimore, Maryland, Charles C Thomas, Publisher, 1935.

Cornejo Bourancle, Jorge: Las momias Incas — trepanaciones craneanas en el antiguo Peru. Actas Inter Cong Americanistas 27, vol. 1: 34-48, Lima, 1940.

Cosgrove, C.B.: A note on a trephined Indian skull from Georgia. Am J Phys Anthropol 13 (2): 353-357, 1929.

Costaeus, Joannis: De igneis medicinae praesidiis. Libro duo. Venice, Robertum Meiettum, 1595.

Crosse-Upcott, A.R.W.: Male circumcision among the Ngindo. J Roy Anthropol Inst 89 pt 2, 169-188, 1959.

Crump, J.A.: Trephining in the South Seas. J Roy Anthropol Inst 31: 167-172, 1901.

Cummins, S.L.: Sub-tribes of the Bahr-el-Ghazal Dinkas. J Anthropol Inst 34: 149-166, 1904.

Daland, Judson: Depressed fracture and trephining of the skull by the Incas of Peru. Ann Med Hist n.s. 7: 550-558, 1935.

Dastugue, J.: Un orifice cranien préhistorique. Bull et Mém, Soc d'Anthropol de Paris 10; 357-363, 1959.

Dauer, A.M. and Karolyi, L.V.: Maganga — ein wissenschaftlicher Film? Medizinhist J 5: 138-144, 1970.

Dawson, Warren R.: Making a mummy. J Egypt Archaeol 13: 40-49, 1927.

——— : The beginnings: Egypt and Assyria. (Clio Medica series) New York, Hafner Publishing Company, 1964.

——— : The Egyptian medical papyri. In Brothwell and Sandison, 1967, 98-111.

Denig, Edwin Thompson: Indian tribes of the Upper Missouri. Ann Rept Bureau of Amer Ethnol 46: 375-628. Washington, Govt. Printing Office, 1930.

Densmore, Frances: Uses of plants by the Chippewa Indians. Ann Rept Bureau of Amer Ethnol 44: 275-397. Washington, Govt. Printing Office, 1928.

Doig, Frederico Kaufmann: Manual de Arqueolgía Peruana. Lima, Ediciones Peisa, 1969.

Driberg, J.H.: The Lango, a Nilotic tribe of Uganda. London, T. Fisher Unwin, Ltd., 1923.

Elkin, A.P.: The Australian Aborigines: how to understand them. Sydney, Angus and Robertson, 1961.

Ella, Samuel: Native medicine and surgery in the South Sea Islands. Med Times and Gazette, London 1: 50-51, 1874.

Ellis, E.S.: Ancient peoples and places; primitive anaesthesia and allied conditions. London, Wm. Heinmann Medical Books, Ltd., 1946.

Ellis, William: Polynesian researches during a residence of nearly six years in the South Sea Islands; including descriptions of the natural history and scenery of the islands — with remarks on the history, mythology, traditions, government, arts, manners and customs of the inhabitants. Vol. 2, London, Fisher Son & Jackson, 1829.

Elsberg, C.A.: The Edwin Smith surgical papyrus on diagnosis and treatment of injuries of the skull and spine 5000 years ago. Ann Med Hist n.s. 3: 271-279, 1931.

Felkin, Robert W.: Notes on labour in Central Africa. Edinburgh Med J 29: 922-930, 1884.

Flack, Isaac Harvey [Harvey Graham]: The story of surgery. New York, Doubleday, Doran & company, Inc., 1939.

Fletcher, Robert: On prehistoric trephining and cranial amulets. U.S. Geog. and Geol. Survey of the Rocky Mountain Region, Contrib to North Amer Ethnol 5. Washington, Govt. Printing Office, 1882.

Forbes, R.J.: Extracting, smelting and alloying. In Singer, Holmyard, and Hall, 1954, 527-599.

Fox, C.E.: The threshold of the Pacific; an account of the social organization, magic and religion of the people of San Cristoval in the Solomon Islands. New York, Alfred A. Knopf, 1925.

Furstenburg, A.C.: Bone regeneration in osteomyelitic defects of the cranium. Trans 36 Ann Meet, Laryngol, Rheum, and Otol Soc for 1930: 434-439, 1930.

Garrison, Fielding H.: An introduction to the history of medicine; with medical chronology, suggestions for study and bibliographic data. Philadelphia and London, W.B. Saunders Company, 1929.

Gibbs, James L. Jr.: Peoples of Africa. New York, Chicago, San Francisco, Toronto, London, Holt, Rinehart and Winston, 1965.

Gillman, Henry: Certain characteristics pertaining to ancient man in Michigan. Ann Rept Smithsonian Inst for 1875: 234-245. Washington, Govt. Printing Office, 1876.

Glanville, S.R.K., ed.: The legacy of Egypt. Chap. 7, "Medicine," by Warren R. Dawson. Oxford, Clarendon Press, 1942.

Gould, George M. and Pyle, Walter L.: Anomalies and curiosities of medicine; being an encyclopedic collection of rare and extraordinary cases, and of the most striking instances of abnormality in all branches of medicine and surgery, derived from an exhaustive research of medical literature from its origin to the present day, abstracted, classified, annotated and indexed. New York, Bell Publishing company, 1956.

Graham, Angus: Surgery with flint. Antiquity 4: 233-237, 1930.

Grinnell, George Bird: The cheyenne Indians, their history and ways of life. Vol. 2. New Haven, Yale Univ. Press, 1923.

Guerini, Vincenzo: A history of dentistry; from the most ancient times until the end of the eighteenth century. Pound Ridge, New York, Milford House, Inc., 1969.

Guiard, Émile: La trépination cranienne chez les néolithiques et chez les primitifs modernes. Paris, Masson et Cie, 1930.

Guthrie, Douglas: A history of medicine. London, Edinburgh, Paris, Melbourne, Toronto and New York, Thomas Nelson and Sons, Ltd., 1945.

Haddon, Alfred C.: The ethnography of the western tribe of Torres Straits. J Roy Anthropol Inst 19: 297-440, 1890.

———— : Head-hunters; black, white and brown. London, Watts & Co., 1932.

Harley, George Way: Native African medicine, with special reference to its practice in the Mano tribe of Liberia. Cambridge, Mass., Harvard Univ. Press, 1941.

Harris, P.G.: Notes on the Dakarkari peoples of Sokoto province, Nigeria. J Roy Anthropol Inst 68: 113-152, 1938.

Harrison, H.S.: Fire making, fuel and lighting. In Singer, Holmyard and Hall, 1954: 216-237.

Harrison, J. Park: On the artificial enlargement of the ear lobe. J Roy Anthropol Inst 2: 190-199, 1873.

Hastings, James, ed.: Encyclopaedia of religion and ethics. Vol. 3. New York, Charles Scribner's Sons, 1913.

Held, G.J.: The Papuas of Waropen. The Hague, Martinus Nijhoff, 1957.

Hilton-Simpson, Melville William: Some Arab and Shawia remedies and notes on the trepanning of the skull in Algeria. J Roy Anthropol Inst 43: 706, 1913.

Hilton-Simpson, M.W.: Arab medicine and surgery; a study of the healing art in Algeria. London, Oxford Univ. Press, 1922.

Hooton, E.A.: Oral surgery in Egypt during the Old Empire. Harvard African Studies I; Cambridge, Mass., Peabody Museum of Harvard University: 29-32, 1917.

Hooton, Earnest A.: The ancient inhabitants of the Canary Islands. Harvard African Studies VII. Cambridge, Mass., Peabody Museum of Harvard University, 1925.

Horsley, Victor: Trephining in the Neolithic period. J Anthropol Inst 17: 100-106, 1888.

Hrdlička, Ales: Trepanation among prehistoric people, especially in America. Ciba Symposia 1 (6): 170-177, 1939.

Jhering, Hermann von: Die Künstliche Deformirung der Zähne. Zeit für Ethnol 14: 213-262, 1882.

Jones, W.H.S., Philosophy and medicine in ancient Greece with an edition of Περὶ ἀρχαίης ἰητρικῆς Bull Hist Med, supp. no. 8, 1946.

Joya, Mock: Mock Joya's things Japanese. Tokyo, Tokyo New Service, Ltd., 1968.

Karsten, Rafael: The civilization of the South American Indians; with special reference to magic and religion. New York, Alfred A. Knopf, 1926.

Kerr, Walter Montagu: The far interior; a narrative of travel and adventure from the Cape of Good Hope across the Zambesi to the lake regions of Central Africa. Boston, Houghton Mifflin and Company, 1886.

Kidd, Dudley: The essential Kafir; London, Adam and Charles Black, 1904.

Kodama, Sakuzaemon: Ainu; historical and anthropologial studies. Sapporo, Japan, Hokkaido Univ. School of Med., 1970.

Landor, A. Henry Savage: In the forbidden land; and account of a journey in Tibet, capture by the Tibetan authorities, imprisonment, torture and ultimate release. Vol. 1. London, William Heinmann, 1898.

Leach, Maria, ed.: Funk and Wagnalls standard dictionary of folklore, mythology and legend. Vol. 1. New York, Funk & Wagnalls Company, 1949.

Lillico, Joan: Primitive blood-letting. Ann Med Hist 2, ser. 3: 133-139, 1940.

Lissowski, F.P.: Prehistoric and early trepanation. In Brothwell and Sandison, 1967, 651, 672.

Livingston, R.W.: The legacy of Greece. Oxford, The Clarendon Press, 1942.

Lumholtz, Carl and Hrdlička, Ales: Trephining in Mexico. Amer Anthropol 10 (12): 389-396, 1897.

Macalister, R.A.S.: A textbook of European archaeology, Vol. 1. The Palaeolithic period. Cambridge, Cambridge Univ. Press, 1921.

MacCurdy, G.G.: Prehistoric surgery — a Neolithic survival. Amer Anthropol n.s. 7: 15-23, 1905.

MacCurdy, George Grant: Surgery among the ancient Peruvians. Art & Archaeol 7: 381-394, 1918.

———— : Human skeletal remains from the highlands of Peru. Am J Phys Anthropol 6 (3): 218-329, 1923.

Macdonald, James: Manners, customs, superstitions and religions of South African tribes. J Anthropol Inst 19: 264-296, 1890.

Macewen, William: The growth of bone; observations on osteogenesis, an experimental inquiry into the development and reproduction of diaphyseal bone. Glasgow, James Maclehose and Sons, 1912.

Majno, Guido: The healing hand; man and wound in the ancient world. Cambridge, Mass., Harvard Univ. Press, 1975.

Major, Ralph H.: A history of medicine. 2 vols. Springfield, Ill., Charles C Thomas, Publisher, 1954.

Malcolm, L.W.G.: Prehistoric and primitive surgery. Nature, Feb. 10, 1934: 200-201.

Margetts, Edward L.: Trepanation of the skull by the medicine-men of primitive cultures with particular reference to present-day native East African practice. In Brothwell and Sandison, 1967: 673-701.

Mason, J. Alden: The ancient civilizations of Peru. Baltimore, Penguin Books, 1968.

Max Müller, W.: Egyptian (in Mythology of All Races, vol. 12) 1-245. Boston, Marshall Jones Company, 1918.

McKenzie, Dan: The infancy of medicine; an enquiry into the influence of folk-lore upon the evolution of scientific medicine. London, Macmillan and Co., Limited, 1927.

Metraux, Alfred: Mourning rites and burial forms of the South American Indians. Amer Indigina 7 (1): 7-44, 1947.

Miklucho-Maclay, N. von: Beright über Operationen Australischer

Eingeborner. Zeit für Ethnol 14: 26-29, 1882.

Milne, John Stewart: Surgical instruments in Greece and Roman times. Oxford, The Clarendon Press, 1907.

Montagu, M.F. Ashley: The origin of subincision in Australia. Oceania 8: 193-207, 1937.

———— : Ritual mutilation among primitive peoples. Ciba Symposia 8 (7): 420-436, 1946.

Moodie, Roy L.: Studies in Palaeopathology; the diseases of the ancient Peruvians and some account of their surgical practices. Surgical Clinics of Chicago 4 (1): 211-231, Feb. 1920(a).

———— : Primitive surgery in ancient Egypt. Surgical Clinics of Chicago 4 (2): 349-358, April 1920(b).

———— : The use of the cautery among neolithic and later primitive peoples. Surgical Clinics of Chicago 4 (4): 851-862, August 1920(c).

———— : The amputation of fingers among ancient and modern primitive peoples and other voluntary mutilations indicating some knowledge of surgery. Surgical Clinics of Chicago 4(6): 1299-1306, December 1920(d).

———— : A variant of the sincipetal T in Peru. Amer J Phys Anthropol 4 (2): 219-222, April-June 1921.

———— : Palaeopathology; an introduction to the study of ancient evidences of disease. Urbana, Ill., Univ. of Illinois Press, 1923.

———— : Prehistoric surgery in New Mexico. Studies in Palaeopathology 24. Am J Surgery n.s. 8 (4): 905-908, 1930.

———— : Studies in Palaeopathology 23: An unusual skull from Pre-Columbian Peru. Amer J Surgery n.s. 8 (4): 903-904, 1930.

Muñiz, Manuel Antonio and McGee, W.J.: Primitive trephining in Peru. Ann Rept Bureau of Amer Ethnol 16: 3-72. Washington, Govt. Printing Office, 1897.

Murdoch, John: Ethnological results of the Point Barrow expedition. Ann Rept Bureau of Amer Ethnol 9: 3-441. Washington, Govt. Printing Office, 1892.

Nordenskiöld, Erland: Modifications in Indian culture through inventions and loans. Goteborg, Elanders Boktryckeri Aktiebolag, 1930.

Oakley, K.P.; Brooke, Winfred M.A.; Kester, A. Roger; and Brothwell, D.R.: Contributions on trephining or trephination in ancient and modern times. Man 59: 93-96, June 1959.

Oppenheim, A. Leo: A cesarian section in the second millenium B.C. J Hist Med 15 (3): 292-294, July 1960.

Ottenberg, Phoebe: The Afikpo Ibo of Eastern Nigeria. In Gibbs 1965: 3-39.

Packard, Francis R.: History of medicine in the United States. Vol. 1. New York and London, Hafner Publishing Company, 1963.

Parry, T. Wilson: Three skulls from Palestine showing two types of primitive surgical holing: being the first skulls exhibiting this phenomenon that have been discovered on the mainland of Asia. Man 36: 170-171, Oct. 1936.

Persson, Ove: A trepanned skull from the Gillhög passage-grave at Barsebak in West Scania (Southern Sweden). Ossa 3/4: 53-61, 1976/1977.

Phillips, E.D.: Greek medicine. London, Thames and Hudson, 1973.

Piggot, Stuart: A trepanned skull of the Beaker period from Dorset and the practice of trepanning in prehistoric Europe. Proc Prehist Soc of East Anglia 6 (3): 112-131, 1940.

————— : Ancient Europe, from the beginnings of agriculture to classical antiquity, a survey. Chicago, Aldine Publishing Co., 1965.

Pindborg, J.J.: Dental mutilation and associated abnormalities in Uganda. Amer J Phys Anthropol 31 (3): 383-389, 1969.

Pollak, Kurt and Underwood, E. Ashforth: The healers: the doctor, then and now. London and Edinburgh, Thomas Nelson, Ltd., 1968.

Powell, Bernard W.: Aboriginal trephination: a case from southern New England? Science 170 (3959): 732-734, 1970.

Radcliffe-Brown, A.R.: The Andaman Islanders. Glencoe, Ill., The Free Press, 1948.

Ranke, Hermann: Medicine and surgery in Ancient Egypt. Bull Hist Med 1: 237-257, 1933.

Rivers, W.H.R.: Medicine, magic and religion: the Fitzpatrick lectures delivered before the Royal College of Physicians of London in 1915 and 1916. London, Kegan Paul, Trench, Trubner & Co., Ltd., 1924.

Rogers, Lambert: The history of craniotomy: an account of the methods which have been practiced and the instruments used for opening the human skull during life. Anns Med Hist 2: 495-514, 1930.

Rogers, Spencer L.: A case of surgical amputation from aboriginal Peru. San Diego Museum of Man, Ethnic Technology Notes 11, 1973.

Rogers, Spencer and Anderson, Arthur J.O.: La terminología anatomica de los Mexicas Precolombinos. Act y Mem 36 Cong Inter de Americanistas 2: 69-76. Seville 1966.

Romero, Javier: Mutilaciones dentarias prehispanicas de Mexico y America en general. Mexico D.F., Inst Nac de Antropol e Hist, 1958.

Roney, James G., Jr.: The occurrence of trephining among the Bakhtiari. Bull Hist Med 28 (5): 489-491, 1954.

Roth, Walter Edmund: An introductory study of the arts, crafts and customs of the Guiana Indians. Ann Rept Bureau of Amer Ethnol 38: 25-720. Washington, Govt. Printing Office, 1924.

Ruffer, Armand: Some recent researches on prehistoric trephining. J Path and Bact 22: 90-104, 1918-1919.

Rytel, Michael M.: Trephinations in ancient Peru. Polish Med Sci Hist 5: 42-45, 1962.

Sahagún, Bernardino de: General history of the things of New Spain. Book 10, The people. Translated by Arthur J.O. Anderson and Charles E. Dibble. Santa Fe, New Mexico, School of American Research and The University of Utah, 1961.

Salaman, Redcliffe: Deformities and mutilations of the face as depicted in the Chiumu pottery of Peru. J Roy Anthropol Inst 69, pt. 1: 109-122, 1939.

Saville, Marshall H.: Pre-Columbian decoration of the teeth in Ecuador; with some account of the occurrence of the custom in other parts of North and South America. Amer Anthropol n.s. 15: 377-394, 1913.

Schadewaldt, Hans: Schädeltrepanationen in Afrika. Medizinhist J 5: 289-298, 1970.

Schapera, I., ed.: The Bantu-speaking tribes of South Africa: an ethnographical survey. London, Routledge & Kegan Paul, Ltd., 1953.

Schultz, Adolph H.: Notes on diseases and healed fractures of wild apes. In Brothwell and Sandison, 1967: 47-55.

Seligman, C.G.: The medicine, surgery and midwifery of the Sinaugolo. J Roy Anthropol Inst 32: 297-304, 1902.

Shapiro, H.L.: Primitive surgery: first evidence of trephining in the Southwest. Nat Hist 27: 266-269, 1927.

Shortt, John: Habits and manners of Mavar tribes of India. Mem Anthropol Soc Lond 3: 201-215, 1867-1868-1869.

Sigerist, Henry E.: A history of medicine, Vol. 1; Primitive and archaic medicine. New York, Oxford Univ. Press, 1951.

Singer, Charles and Underwood, E. Ashworth: A short history of medicine. 2nd ed. Oxford, Clarendon Press, 1962.

Singer, Charles, Holmyard, E.J. and Hall, A.R., eds.: A history of technology. New York and London, Oxford Univ. Press, 1954.

Smith, G. Elliot: The most ancient splints. Brit Med J., March 28, 1908: 723-734.

Smith, Harlan I.: Trephined aboriginal skulls from British Columbia and

Washington. Am J Phys Anthropol 7 (4) 447-452, 1924.

Söderström, J.: Die Rituellen Fingerverstummellungen in der Südsee und in Australien. Zeit für Ethnol 70 (1/2): 24-47, 1938.

Spencer, Baldwin: Native tribes of the northern territory of Australia. London, Macmillan and Co., Limited, 1914.

Spencer, Baldwin and Gillen, F.J.: The Arunta: a study of Stone Age people. Two vols. London, Macmillan and Co., Limited, 1927.

Squier, E. George: Peru: incidents of travel and exploration in the land of the Incas. New York, Harper & Brothers, Publishers, 1877.

Stannus, Hugh Stannus: The Wayo of Nyasaland. Harvard African Studies, vol. 3, 229-372. Cambridge, Mass., Peabody Museum of Harvard University, 1922.

Steinbock, R. Ted: Paleopathological diagnosis and interpretation: bone diseases in ancient human populations. Springfield, Ill., Charles C Thomas, Publisher, 1976.

Stewart, T.D.: Deformity, trephining, and mutilation in South American Indian skeletal remains. In Steward 1950, Handbook of South American Indians, vol. 6: 43-48, 1950.

———— : The significance of osteitis in ancient Peruvian trephining. Bull Hist Med 30: 293-320, 1956.

———— : Stone Age skull surgery. A general reivew with emphasis on the New World. Ann Rept Smithsonian Inst for 1957, 469-491. Washington, Govt. Printing Office, 1958.

———— : Are supra-inion depressions evidence of prophylactic trephination? Bull Hist Med 50: 414-434, 1976.

———— : The Neanderthal skeletal remains from Shanidar Cave, Iraq: a summary of findings to date. Proc Amer Philos Soc 121 (2): 121-165, April 1977.

Stone, Eric: Medicine among the American Indians. New York, Hafner Publishing Company, 1962.

Sumner, William Graham and Keller, Albert Galloway: The science of society. Four vols. New Haven, Yale Univ. Press, 1928.

Swanton, John R.: Religious beliefs and medical practices of the Creek Indians. Ann Rept Bureau of Amer Ethnol 42: 473-672. Washington, Govt. Printing Office, 1928.

Tello, Julio C.: Prehistoric trephining among the Yauyos of Peru. Proc Inter Cong of Americanists 18th session, part 1: 75-83. London 1913.

Thomas, N.W.: Natives of Australia. London, Archibald Constable and Company, Ltd., 1906.

Thompson, C.J.S.: The history and evolution of surgical instruments. New York, Schuman's 1942.

Thorndike, Lynn: A history of magic and experimental science during the first thirteen centuries of our era. Vol. 1. New York and London, Columbia Univ. Press, 1923.

Torday, E. and Joyce, T.A.: Notes on the ethnography of the Ba-Yaka. J Anthrop Inst 36: 39-59, 1906.

Trepanation in Cornish miners. Ciba Symposia 1 (6): 197, Sept. 1939.

Turnbull, Colin M.: Initiation among the Ba Mbuti Pygmies of the central Ituri. J Roy Anthropol Inst 87, pt. 2: 191-216, Dec. 1957.

Turner, G.A.: Circumcision amongst natives. Med J So Africa 10 (8): 133-138, 1915.

Vélez López, Lizardo: La cirugia del cráneo en los vasos del Peru precolombino. Actas y Trabajos del cong de Americanistas 27, vol. 1: 27-34, Lima 1940.

Vogel, Virgil J.: American Indian medicine. Norman, Okla., Univ. of Oklahoma Press, 1970.

Wakefield, E.G. and Dellinger, Samuel G: Possible reasons for trephining the skull in the past. Ciba Symposia 1 (6): 166-169, Sept. 1939.

Wangensteen, Owen H.: Some early Greek heroes of medicine: the training of surgeons and some post-Hunterian schools of surgery. J Hist Med 34 (2): 211-222, April 1979.

Wangensteen, Owen and Wangensteen, Sarah D.: The rise of surgery from empiric craft to scientific discipline. Minneapolis, Univ. of Minnesota Press, 1978.

Wells, Calvin: Bones, bodies and disease: evidences of disease and abnormality in early man. New York, Frederick A. Praeger, 1964.

Wölfel, d.J.: Die Trepanation: Studien über Ursprung, Zusammenhänge und kulturelle Zugehörigkeit der Trepanation. Anthropos 20: 1-50, 1925.

Wollaston, A.F.R.: Pygmies & Papuans: the Stone Age to-day in Dutch New Guinea. New York, Sturgis and Walton Company, 1912.

NAME INDEX

123

SUBJECT INDEX